2 Da)

By Dr.

An effortless weight loss process you can do together

"Dr. Christensen is an extraordinary author. Simply put, his research on how to give yourself a 2-day gift of wellness is priceless. This gift will keep on giving for the rest of your life, with his unique process of utilizing your "Triple 'R' days". – Debra Thomas, Integrative Nutrition Health Coach (INHC)

"I found Dr. Michael's book, *2 Day Gift of Wellness* to be exceptionally well written, a quick read and very easy to understand. Dr. Michael achieves two primary goals. He clearly demonstrates the downfalls of most diets, at the same time giving the reader an alternative that targets wellness which normally achieves weight loss as a side-effect. The virtue of his process is that it has been proven to be sustainable which is difficult in most diets. I recommend this book to anyone who wants to lose weight and keep it off, while improving their health, their energy and their state of mind." – John Berish

"A must read for folks who've been unsuccessful with traditional diet plans, or anyone seeking better health and wellness. Dr. Christensen explains why those traditional diet plans ultimately fail and offers a path to better health and wellness through his UdP™ process. He lays out UdP's eight basic principles in clear, easy to understand language and includes real world examples of his clients' experiences and successes, along with sample menus and journaling. For folks like me, who must travel internationally across many time zones, his tips for achieving UdP success on the road are invaluable. – Phil C., MD-11 Captain

"I started to measure my success in ways other than just weight loss. I noticed that I was feeling more grounded, more at peace, in spite of the fact that there were some very stressful things happening during this period of my life." - Christie Z.

"Without my partner, I would never been able to attempt this process in my current state. My wife has been completely supportive, and she has been an excellent example of how the process should work." - Dave Z.

"I was surprised at how easy the process is ... how effortless it has been to make the necessary changes. How easily I have embraced [the UdP] as something I will continue for the rest of my life. Weight is literally falling off without much effort. When I start walking again, it will really start coming off. I have lost 21 pounds since March! I have lost almost 4 pounds the 1st week of vacation - unheard of!" -Karen D.

"I have good energy, haven't had any heartburn since I started [the UdP]. My weight is dropping at a steady pace. This process is sustainable long term. I realized when I stepped on the scales a few days ago at 235 lbs., that's almost 20 lbs. lost in 6 weeks. - Larry C.

"I noticed my clothes fit better. Trying on wedding dresses was fun! The gal helping me even told me I didn't need to wear the Spanx I had on. I didn't feel like I had to suck in my gut! Thank you!" - Cheri C.

"After my first Triple R day™ of the week, I finally slept great and woke up feeling like I was actually rested for the first time in a long time." - Pam W.

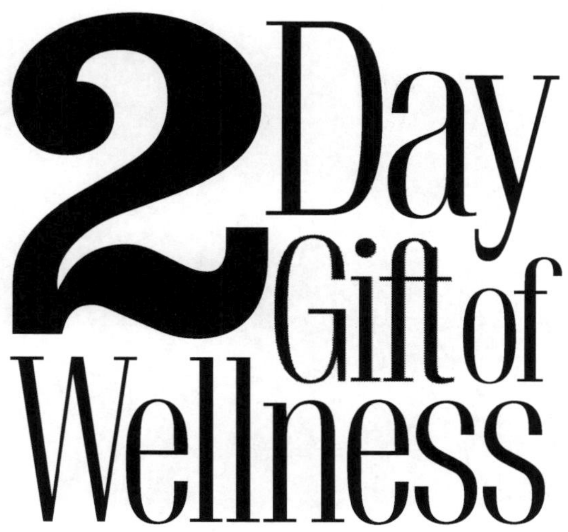

An effortless weight loss process
you can do together

Dr. Michael Christensen

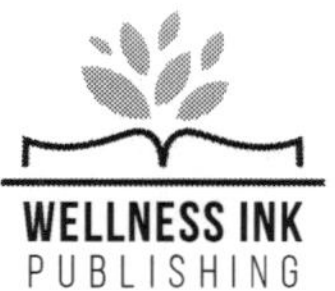

2 Day Gift of Wellness

An effortless weight loss process you can do together

Wellness Ink Publishing: www.WellnessInk.com

First Printing January 2017
Printed in the United States.
Designed by Victoria Valentine
Interior photos by Victoria Brown

ISBN: 978-0-9734734-7-6 (paper)
ISBN:978-0-9734734-8-3 (ebook)

Contact:
DrMichael@2dayGift.com

www.2dayGift.com

Attention: Quantity discounts and customized versions are available for bulk purchases. For permission requests or quantity discounts, please email Dr. Michael Christensen.

Dedication

For my Mom, Winnie Mae Christensen,
my wife, Victoria, and our children.

In different ways, my life began
when I met them.

A Note to Readers

This book is not intended to be a substitute for talking to your physician. It is for informational purposes only. The book does not concentrate on weight loss, but on reaching an ideal weight through healthy lifestyle changes. In this regard the author and publisher encourage you to use the information in this book with health care professionals, personal trainers, and nutritionists. They are perfect team members in your quest for increased wellness and a longer life. Everyone is different and you should consult with your team before beginning this or any program to tailor it to your individual needs. The author and publisher expressly disclaim responsibility for any adverse effects that may result for the use, misuse, or application of the information contained in this book.

Table of Contents

Foreword

What a coincidence. Nearly 30 years had passed since I met Mike Christensen. I was an Air Force instructor pilot and Mike was a recent graduate from the United States Air Force Academy and was entering USAF pilot training. I had the distinguished privilege of "soloing" Mike in his first high-performance jet. That was in the 1980s. Later in 2012 we would meet again. This time, I took on the role of Chair of his doctoral dissertation committee. What is coincidental about our second meeting is that due to the amount of time that had passed, we did not initially recognize each other. So there we were working together again, clueless about our earlier relationship. I don't recall which of the two of us finally came to the conclusion we had met in our Air Force days, however I must say it was quite a meaningful experience to become aware of our earlier flying days together.

Looking back as Dr. Christensen's instructor pilot in the Air Force and again as Chair of his dissertation committee, I can say with pronounced sincerity that Mike produces outstanding work. He makes no claims that go unsubstantiated. Nor does he insinuate to his readers something other than scientifically-derived and well-founded fact. Simply stated, Mike knows what he's talking about. Take time with this book. Make it a part of your *process of living*. Go the distance. And I have a hunch, you will be happy you did.

Now, a few words about the book itself.

The book you are about to read – and study and use as a reference for years to come – was written by a highly creative and talented author. Whether you are new to the notion of losing weight and becoming healthier, or one of many who have searched extensively for effective diets, you will find this book invaluable.

2 Day Gift of Wellness is unique for one highly important reason, process. In this book, you will learn to shift your attention away from *what* you are eating to *how* you are eating. In psychological terms, you will experience a *content to process shift*. Dr. Christensen's Ultimate diet Process™ gently yet effectively shifts your attention away from calorie counting and toward what he calls a synergy of the mind, body, and spirit for healthy living. Additionally, his ingenious approach leads to increased creativity, a longer life, and almost accidental weight loss. *Accidental* being the key word here.

Some of the important concepts Dr. Christensen addresses – my top 5 if you will – include 1) the secret fat connection, 2) eating when you're hungry, 3) the Triple R day, 4) UdP buddies, and 5) journaling via Triple R questions. Of course, there are a quite a few more concepts to choose from, I just have my favorites. I recommend developing your own list of gems from the array offered throughout the book.

This book is highly practical. It is certainly easy-to-read, interesting, and immediately useful to the reader by way of important stories and useful tips and practices. Additionally, ample theoretical background is provided and thoroughly substantiates

Dr. Christensen's approach. *2 Day Gift of Wellness* is a must for every person whose life involves focus on health and exceptional well-being. I predict this book will become an important resource to those interested in a happy, healthy, and well-balanced life.

– *Michael J Vandermark, PhD*
President, Vandermark and Associates, Inc.
Author of *Life's Wake-up Call: the Content to Process Shift*

A note from Joseph Patrick Santiago, MD

People never say, "I want to improve my heart health for two months," but they treat weight loss as a temporary situation.

A friend of mine, who is also a patient, used to weigh 350 lbs. Over the course of five years he lost about half that weight to get down to 170-180 pounds, and has kept the weight off so far. He simply ate better and exercised regularly. He made a comment that I'd never thought of in sixteen years of primary care private practice.

It was a remarkable insight: "For every pound of physical weight I lost, I had to lose two pounds of mental weight. I had to rethink and retool the way I lived my life before I could get physically healthier."

In sixteen years of private practice I've never seen anyone who had weight loss surgery keep the weight off permanently. All the patients I've seen who lost weight and kept it off were able to achieve their goals by creating new habits and lifestyle changes. It's the sustainability that matters.

So many people are okay with the idea of taking medication for the rest of their lives, but for some reason don't think of eating better and exercising as equally important to long term health. Nobody comes to my office asking me to reduce their risk of a heart attack for just three months. But that's what people do when they don't stick with eating right and being physically active. I've told my patients that weight loss isn't just eating healthier food and being fit. It's a conscious effort to retool the way you live your life. That's why this book is such as gift to anyone who wants to get well and stay well.

– Joseph Patrick Santiago, MD

Introduction

Why I wrote this book

Like everyone else I know, I've been on diets throughout my life. I was never obese but I always thought I was a little heavier than I should be. When I look back at pictures in high school and college, I think how skinny I was, but I don't remember feeling that way at the time.

When I dieted, especially in the military, I'd lose just enough to squeak below the maximum weight allowed. Two weeks later, I'd be over that weight with an added five pounds. I'd stay that way for the next year or two and then start all over again. So from the very beginning I felt that dieting doesn't really work. But I wasn't that much above my ideal weight so I didn't worry about it.

I had several close friends and family members who went through surgery to lose weight. It was traumatic for them and shocking for everyone who witnessed it. We watched them endure this surgery and then feel violently ill afterwards. They couldn't eat anything because their stomachs were stapled, and they'd throw up every few hours. They did lose the weight, but it was a very harrowing experience. The distressing thing was that even with their stapled stomachs, they gained the weight back within a year or so.

So I kept thinking that something was missing from this whole process. I heard absurd statements like, "If you eat yogurt with probiotics, you'll double your weight loss." I suspected that couldn't possibly be true and I wanted to investigate.

One day a colleague mentioned that his teenaged daughter was having issues with bulimia. I thought, "This really doesn't make any sense. I'm going to explore and figure out what happened."

I came across an old book my brother had given me several years before about the musings of a Chinese philosopher. *Translations from the Chinese* was published in 1927 but the first copyrights were in the early 1900s. One of the musings really stood out to me as I started this journey. It reminded me of how the diet industry treats the truth. It's called:

The Truth Will Condemn You

It's a mark of extreme youth to believe
That telling the whole truth is always useful.
Truth is not a diet
but a condiment.

—The Old Mandarin

While I'm not a medical doctor, I am well versed in reading and understanding research studies. So I decided to take a deep dive into the research without the bias associated with the individual disciplines of medicine or nutrition.

It seemed to me that each field was stuck in its own narrow tower and didn't cross over. I wanted to review the research through a variety of disciplines including medicine, nutrition, exercise science, straight weight loss, vegetarian and vegan diets, meat-only diets, metabolic adaption, fad diets, high protein, low-carb, high-carb, low-fat, intermittent fasting, when to eat, calorie reduction diets, and obesity data.

There are thousands of different ways to approach weight loss, so I decided to hit them from many different angles. I used only peer-reviewed research and not popular health or nutrition magazines because they tend to be sensationalist. When I went back to look at the studies, their reports weren't what the actual studies said. That's why I decided to write this book.

I can see the forest, not for the trees, but for the living organic entity that it is.

UdP – The Ultimate diet Process™

UdP stands for the **Ultimate diet Process**. It's different because I looked at it from a different perspective. Everyone is blessed with certain innate talents and abilities, and mine include the ability to peer through the clutter and come up with central ideas, seeing the trees for the forest, if you will. But my talent is really more than that. I can see with clarity the entire forest, the stream coming in and the river flowing out. I can see the subtle changes of the leaves and bushes that make the forest a living organic system.

I noticed that focusing on weight loss distorted the picture. So I decided to research a concept called ideal weight, which we'll talk about later. The UdP would be a synergy of all the research I've done. It would take the focus off weight loss and put it squarely onto healthy habits, where ideal weight or weight loss are a natural result.

I learned that the body is constantly attacked and stressed by the environment. Even the digestive process is stressful. When you look at nutrition instead of looking at what we eat, it's really looking at what your body wants to eat to get the nutrition it requires. It truly is a unique personalized approach to ideal weight and healthy living.

UdP synergizes the mind, body, and spirit for healthy living, increased creativity, and a longer life, all the while creating weight loss, almost accidently.

A good decision is based on knowledge and not on numbers. – Plato

---

My story

Throughout this book, you'll read stories of my clients who have been through the Ultimate diet Process (UdP). In this section, I'll write a little about my experience living the UdP lifestyle.

I wrote this book because I had very discouraging results with several popular diets. I am an international Boeing 777 Captain with a large American commercial airline. My job requires that I maintain a healthy weight. But like most people I had gained and lost the same 10–20 pounds many times in my life, always putting on an extra 5 pounds for good measure. I'd heard all the standard diet advice, such as "eat less, exercise more." Intuitively I knew that wasn't true.

I decided I needed to do some in-depth research into the diet industry. I graduated with my Doctor of Management degree in 2015. The experience of understanding peer-reviewed scientific studies gave me an idea. What if I did a deep dive into the diet industry, throwing aside all I thought I knew, and going where the data led?

What I found was that most of what I read in popular magazines, US Government recommendations, and online was wrong. The studies just didn't support the conclusions. For example, when I would ask friends or colleagues about weight loss they would often say that all I have to do is exercise more and eat less. This is the old calorie-in/ calorie-out approach. One popular diet program gave additional points for working out. The research however, showed a different result. (Forthergill, et al., 2016; Lucan & DiNicolantonio, 2015; Monteiro & Cannon, 2015; Rosenbaum, Hirsch, Gallagher, Leibel, 2008).

My Masters' Degree from USC was in Systems Management, so looking at weight loss from a holistic approach made sense to me. From my psychology degree at the United States Air Force Academy, I knew the mind had great control over the body, but could not maintain its hold indefinitely.

With these tools I did lengthy research into everything related to weight loss. Using my unique skills to visualize the entire system that occurs in wellness, I looked at respected current studies that were peer-reviewed and scientifically sound. I did not use any popular magazines or internet blogs. I went right to the data. I used research conducted since 2014, unless the study was particularly relevant (ground breaking). What I found was amazing.

The body has a weight "set point" that it guards with all its energy. This set point is the pivot for the yo-yo dieting syndrome.

For instance, research shows the body has a "set point" that it thinks is the correct weight based on a number of internal systems and receptacles. This set point has no bearing to what current fashion dictates, or even what fad diet you are on. It is based on age, weight, stress, illness, genetics, and evolution (Aamodt, 2016; Pontzer, 2015). The body will do whatever it needs to get back to that weight. Because the body is an open system, it reacts to ANYTHING the mind makes it do.

If the mind restricts calories, the body becomes more efficient with the use of calories. The body, without the mind's approval or knowledge, restricts the energy use during non-peak times to make up for this reduction, even after you have started exercising. The body also seems to make fat out of air. The human body truly is amazing.

So, using all the data I accumulated from the studies, I designed a process to take advantage of my knowledge. I first tested the concepts I developed on myself and lost 26 pounds in 4 months without exercising. I accomplished this while flying internationally and I wasn't starving myself. Just the opposite, and I increased my energy levels and creativity.

My first officer (co-pilot) witnessed my effortless weight loss while on layovers in China, Japan, Singapore, and Malaysia. He didn't say much during the trip, but when I was looking for a test group, he insisted I let him participate. Here is a note he wrote after 11 weeks on the program. You can read an expanded version of Larry's journey in Chapter 11, UdP on the road - the travelers' guide.

Larry's story

Elk season began in Idaho this week. For me and my hunting partner, this meant 4:30 am wake ups, hiking 3-5 miles in the morning at elevations from 7500-9500 feet with 30 pounds of gear, taking a mid-day nap, and then doing it over again in the afternoon until dark at 8:30 pm.

By the time we get back to camp and eat dinner, we are left with about 6 hours of sleep before the next 4:30 am alarm goes off. In seasons past, after a couple of days we would have to take a morning or an afternoon off to recover from exhaustion.

This year, after 11 weeks of the UdP, I started the season about 10-15 pounds lighter than last year and with the same amount of pre-season working out. I noticed on the very first day how much better I felt hiking up the hills. Climbing was easier, I did not get as winded as usual, and I had good energy all day.

My hunting partner is 5 years younger, 80 pounds lighter, and works out a lot, but I've been kicking his butt climbing hills this year.

Larry's story is not unusual. The secret was discovering that weight was just a number. So my research began to center around holistic wellness. I looked for activities in which the research showed weight loss as a by-product, not the intended result. But the activities had to be beneficial to health. By concentrating on getting healthier using specific behaviors and activities, I discovered you could live a longer, healthier life at the ideal weight your body sets for you.

The UdP is a diet killer, not a killer diet!

My goal was to develop a diet killer – a process where the reason you eat is more important than what you eat. The UdP isn't a content-driven program. You decide what you eat. It is designed to be sustainable. You will never diet again, because there is no need to. A core principle is to eat when you are hungry. You eat what you enjoy and discover foods that are good for your body, along with other foods you might want to limit or cut out.

You decide which two days to devote to activities that reduce or eliminate stress and allow your body to repair itself. You decide what type of exercise you want to do. None of these actions alone promote weight loss. But together, along with a few more specific activities, they increase your wellbeing and allow your body to relax and not store as much fat.

You see, fat is a rainy day fund for your body. If your mind and your body are in sync, your body will automatically and effortlessly lose fat. But you have to follow the plan exactly. As Einstein said, you can't keep doing things the same way and expect different results.

They All Fall Down

I've built three homes,
One worse than the other.
But one final try today.

I have the plans, but I'm proficient,
I alter to suit my needs;
Then watching, disbelieving, as #4 dissolves.

©2016 From the upcoming book *Ballet in a Coal Mine*: the musings of a Dr. Captain, publishing date January 2017.

I've done the research and now you can follow this new plan. Don't fall back into old ways that don't work. Involving a buddy, partner, or family member will significantly improve your chances of success. This plan is simple, but not always easy at first. It requires a paradigm shift from everything you've heard. You can hire one of our mentors to help, but ultimately you make the commitment to be a better you. Even with a partner, you travel the road independently. Each of you can eat whatever you enjoy. There is no requirement to eat or avoid any specific foods.

How will your journey go? I can't say. Most of us need to lose weight, and if you follow the plan you probably will. But remember, weight is just a number. Ultimately it is meaningless. It is wellness that counts. It's getting your body and mind in sync. It's about increasing your health.

As a pilot I am required to have a flight physical every 6 months. During my last checkup, my flight doctor noticed my weight loss and asked about it. I was a little shy about sharing my system with a physician. He waived off my concern saying, "Doctors don't know about wellness." Then he took my blood pressure, which was 107/79. Next he took my pulse, which was in the low 50's. He knew I wasn't on any medications, and at my age he thought that was amazing. After asking a few more questions, he said he wanted to buy my book as soon as it was published.

The UdP is simple, but you have to follow the plan exactly as developed – no short cuts.

The unbelievable part of the UdP journey is that it is sustainable. Change comes slowly and permanently. I noticed I didn't require any allergy medicine, even though we've had one of the worst allergy seasons in memory. I couldn't remember the last time my plantar fasciitis acted up. My prostate had shrunk and I swear my gray hair started getting darker. One client noted she hadn't had irritable bowel syndrome for over a month. Another client with acid reflux suddenly realized he didn't have that anymore. All these people lost significant amounts of weight, but the real benefit was their health. Their bodies had begun to rejuvenate.

Everyone remarked that their clothes fit better than the weight loss should allow. The body changes and digests the unwanted fat before it shows on the scale. One client wanted to lose that last stubborn 5 pounds. I explained that this is about wellness, not reaching a target weight. She committed to the process, and started fitting into clothes she never thought she would. By week three she was engaged. She lost 6 pounds the first month and genuinely enjoyed shopping for her wedding dress. There are stories like this throughout the book.

This book has been a labor of love. While writing it, I've enjoyed being healthier, with more energy and unbelievable creativity. I hope and pray that this book is the beginning of your new, healthier life. No more diets! Enjoy life, and live deliberately.

Take advantage of the UdP

If you're reading this book, I'm assuming there are things you'd like to change in your general health or your weight. Like most people, you've probably tried a series of diets, only to be disappointed as the weight came back on, most likely even more than before. In this book, I'll give you new strategies to achieve the health you've always wanted, along with weight loss as a side-effect, if that's what you want.

This book is organized into 3 parts:

Part 1

- You'll learn about the diet industry's dirty secrets, so you'll discover, once and for all, why you can't maintain the weight you struggle so hard to lose.
- We'll dive into the UdP program, and set you up with the 8 Principles of UdP Wellness, so you have a framework to be healthy in today's world.

Part 2

- You'll be putting the UdP into action. We'll go into detail about what and when to eat, how to create a sustainable eating plan for yourself, and how to benefit from the Triple R day™, which is the heart of our program.

• You'll get the nuts and bolts of every aspect of the program, to set you up for success. You'll also be reading stories of people who have been thru the UdP, and love it so much that they plan to continue for the rest of their lives.

Part 3

• You'll get resources, such as sample menus, questions to answer, and sample journal pages.

With the solutions in this book, you'll learn to harness the power of a program that is based on the best scientific evidence to date, not the sensationalist stories that make the news, only to fade into oblivion the next day. You deserve to have the healthiest and most productive and enjoyable life possible, don't you?

— *Dr. Michael Christensen*

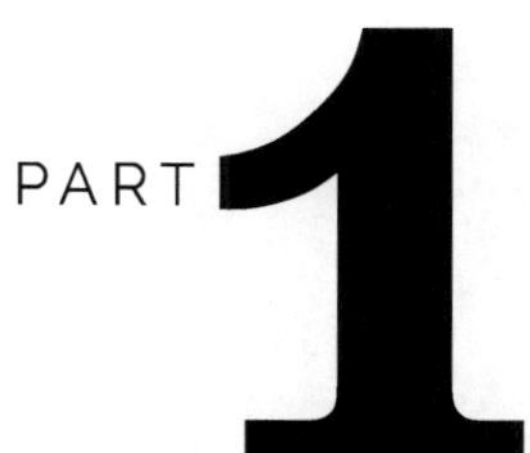

PART 1

From Fat and Stressed to Weight Loss as a Side Effect

CHAPTER 1

Show me the money

The diet industry's dirty secrets

Show me the money! That's what I wanted to know about the diet industry. According to Markets and Markets, a leading research firm, the global weight loss and diet-management products and services market is worth over $671 billion a year.

In contrast, a significant portion of the world's population is close to, or at, starvation levels. I found this perplexing. Borrowing a phrase from the movie Jerry Maguire, "Show me the money," I wanted to research where the money is. I found out that the industry is basically content-oriented, which means focusing on which foods to eat or how much, because there's lots of money to be made.

The global weight loss industry is worth more than $670,000,000.00 a year.

The word "diet" actually comes from two different sources. The Latin and French source of the word is *dieta*, which means daily food allowance. That makes sense when you think of diet programs such as Weight Watchers™, which are based on how much you eat. You have a calorie or point-count to make sure you don't eat more than a specific amount.

The other root of the word diet is from the Greek word, *diaita*, which means "meaning of life." That's closer to what we're looking at. Examples include the Mediterranean diet, and vegetarian or raw food diets which are content-specific. You have to eat a specific group of foods, and avoid others. My beginning research explained the two types of diets, but not *why* we diet.

Most people these days are constantly dieting or are starting diets over and over again. It never seems to end. We diet for many reasons, including physical, psychological, emotional and cultural. Marketing plays a huge role. The global diet market is almost a trillion-dollar-a-year industry, so they have a vested interest in keeping us on the diet roller coaster. The weight loss industry includes fitness, nutrition, health, technology, wellness, supplements, and much more.

They keep that golden goose fat by convincing us to keep buying more health-related items such as diet books and programs, gym memberships, Fitbits, scales, clothes, bicycles, treadmills, running shoes, and yoga mats.

Two dirty secrets about dieting

The industry has two dirty secrets about dieting they don't want you to know. The first secret is the psychological aspect. They know we human beings are insecure and therefore vulnerable to advertisements and suggestions. Marketing preys on our insecurities. We're told we can never be thin enough, and that thin people are more popular and successful. But that's only part of the story.

The second secret is that the diet industry knows dieting doesn't work in the long run. Not only does it not work, but we consistently gain back the weight and add a few extra pounds for good measure.

Most credible diets work in the short run because they are content-driven. You reduce what you eat, and you lose weight. But ultimately it's not sustainable because you have a life to live and you can't keep up with the activities that helped you lose the weight.

By constantly reinforcing our insecurities and developing new diets and products, the diet industry creates a limitless supply of people who want solutions. It really is quite a brilliant scheme if it weren't for the fact that we're talking about people's lives and health.

The diet success stories you hear are a bit like doing your taxes. Somebody will tell you about all the different exemptions they took and how much money they saved, but they never tell you that they got audited a month later, and how bad it was. They only tell you the good side.

Dieting is like taxes – you do it every year, you hate it, every year its more, and it never ends.

That's what happens with dieting. People will tell you, "This diet was great. I lost so much weight." They neglect to tell you that they gained it all back and packed on 10 more pounds. You witness this with your friends and family, but on TV you never see the whole story. And that's what perpetuates the myth that diets work to keep you thin.

The Biggest Losers TV show is a great example of how the second part of the story never gets told, because most of the participants gained most of their weight back (Fothergill, et al, 2016). But it's worse than that.

Dieting can cause harm. There are consequences to constantly dieting, physically and emotionally. That's why all the plans have disclaimers telling you to see your doctor before beginning the program. They have to protect you from the content of their plans which often feed into eating disorders such as anorexia nervosa, bulimia nervosa, or binge eating. In a nutshell, the reason diets don't work long-term is that we fight against our own nature (Aamodt, S., 2016). Our minds fight our bodies, which fight our spirits.

Back in the hunter-gatherer days, we formed groups to hunt prey and forage for food. We only ate what we caught or found. Food was hard to get, and no one was overeating. As we aged, we became less efficient at hunting and gathering. Research speculates that for genetic reasons, based on natural selection (Neil, et al, 1998; Pontzer, et al, 2012), we gain weight as we get older because our metabolism slows down to conserve calories. We're counting on other people to feed us, and may be getting less to eat. So as we age we are naturally inclined to store extra weight.

Today, especially in developed nations, we're a knowledge culture. We don't have to chase a bison and hunt it with a gun or a spear. We use money as a means of catching food. We tend to grow wealthier as we age, and at the same time we are likely to exercise less, without decreasing our food intake.

Instead, many of us eat more and more. So we have two things working against us: the freedom and ability to pick up food any time we want it, and the body's natural tendencies to hold onto weight as we grow older.

What works and what doesn't in weight loss

Your body knows when you're under stress before your mind is even aware of it. It knows when organs are injured or things are going wrong inside you before you feel the effects.

We can learn a lot by looking at what happens when we gain weight back. For instance, we know that after five years, 41% of dieters gain more weight than they lost, no matter how hard they try. Why does that happen? We know that dieters are more likely to become obese than people who have never dieted. In studies where one identical twin dieted and the other didn't, the one who dieted was twice as likely to become overweight than the other one (Dulloo, & Montani, 2015). And women who diet are three times as likely to become obese than those who don't.

Your body knows a lot that it's not telling you.

We also have to understand that exercise is not really a weight loss mechanism because your body has ways of making up for the calories you burn during a workout (Hobkins, et al, 2014; Lucan, S. C., & DiNicolantonio, 2015; Pontzer, et al, 2015).

Counselling doesn't seem to be the answer either. One study from the Journal of Obesity took two groups of people who had lost 10 to 20 pounds. They divided the group in half. One half had monthly counseling, similar to what some of the popular diet plans offer. The other had no counseling. After a year, both groups had regained the same amount of weight. So we know that counselling is not the solution.

So what is the answer?

The next chapter reveals a paradigm shift that lets you work with your body's natural processes. You'll understand how to create wellness, with weight loss or maintaining an ideal weight as a happy side-effect.

CHAPTER 2

The UdP

From content to process – A paradigm shift

Eat this. Don't eat that. You hear this constantly in the media, and in diet books and plans. Most diets are content-based, which means they tell you what kind of food you can or can't eat. They also restrict the amount you eat. They might have points or tell you to eat a specific number of certain kinds of foods, or to reduce your calories by 20% every day. That's content-driven.

A *process* is the way you do something. An example of a process might be picking up rocks. Once you learn how to pick up rocks and put them into a box, you can pick up anything. It could be logs or sticks. You learn the process of picking things up, and as things change, you adapt your process to picking up new objects.

The UdP, or Ultimate diet Process, is process-driven. It requires a paradigm shift. That means going from the content-driven weight loss programs you're used to, to something completely different.

The most notable paradigm shift occurred back in 1543 when Nicolaus Copernicus theorized that the sun was actually the center

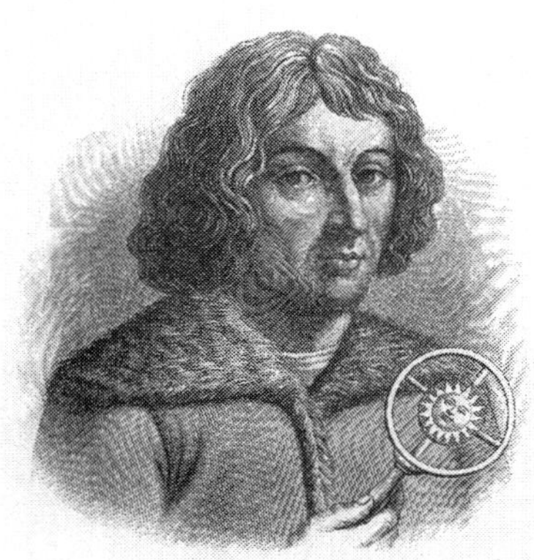
Nicolaus Copernicus

of the universe. Up until that point, everyone believed the earth was the center of the universe. Copernicus looked at all the scientific data and couldn't make the numbers work with the earth as the center. So he decided to shift his view to the sun. Lo and behold, it all began to make sense. Even with overwhelming evidence, it still took 200 years for the scientific community to make that paradigm shift.

Similarly, when we talk about process versus content for weight loss, we're looking at losing weight not as a specific goal but as the by-product of healthy living. Although we use it as a data point, the aim is not to reach a specific number on the scale. That makes the UdP the antidote to commercial diets that are not sustainable, because it works on what your body naturally wants to do instead of fighting your basic nature.

Make the paradigm shift from content (what I eat) to process (how I eat.)

As we touched on earlier, excess weight was not an issue for most of human history. Only wealthy people were fat, and they were envied because they had enough to eat when most people barely had enough food to survive. During the hunter-gatherer days, we could only eat what we could either catch or find. Food was often scarce, so our bodies developed adapting mechanisms such as decreasing our metabolism to keep us from starving to death.

These days we have the opposite problem in the Western world. There's plenty of food available, to the point where many people are obese. So we've created the diet industry to solve the problem. Most diets are based on reducing calories or restricting certain kinds of foods. But by pretending there is some kind of starvation crisis, we unintentionally cause our bodies stress by overriding the normal desire to eat.

Your body's set point

Your body wants you to be a certain weight, based on what it knows and feels. This is called a set point. It tries to maintain equilibrium through the hormones and enzymes that regulate your metabolic rate (Aamodt, 2016). This process is called metabolic adaptation and it persists over time, causing weight to return after a diet (Fothergill, et al, 2016). This includes whether food is processed through the liver and stored as fat, or used right away for fuel, partly based on the amount of stress you feel.

But the body is like the tortoise that always wins the race. It's slow-acting and long-lasting, which is why the standard commercial diets aren't sustainable. The brain can overcome the body momentarily while it's thinking about it. But as soon as it forgets, the body takes over and stores the fat it thinks it needs. When you put your body under stress by reducing your calories, it actually wants to save even more calories, which is why we gain that extra five pounds every time we diet.

This metabolic adaption, which is rooted in genetics based on natural selection, has positive effects (Neel, 1998; Pontzer, 2015). For instance, in 1990 a few days after Iraq invaded Kuwait, I was deployed indefinitely, to Saudi Arabia. I only had 12 hours' notice and couldn't tell my family where I was going. I was one of the first 100 military personnel to be deployed.

I stayed in Saudi Arabia for 5 months. I worked 12 hour shifts with no days off. I ate at the military chow hall or the meals ready-to-eat (MREs) that were provided. Both were very high in calories. Towards the end, we'd make a midnight run off base to pick up shawarmas, a local type of lamb pita, also very high in calories.

I had no time to exercise, so of course I must have gained weight. But no, I actually lost about 25 pounds, effortlessly. That was the first time I ate what I enjoyed and lost weight without trying. After my recent deep dive into weight loss, I now understand the mechanics of what was going on.

Have you ever heard of anyone committing suicide by holding their breath? It can't happen. The body always wins over the mind.

My unconscious mind understood the danger I was in. So, without my conscious thought or physical activity, my body used available fat to strengthen my muscles and heal my body. My unconscious mind and body were preparing me for battle. The change was so gradual, I didn't notice until I returned home and saw photos of me in a local newspaper giving a talk about what it was like "over there."

The UdP is a process to take advantage of the body and mind's ability to work together - subconsciously. The UdP restricts calories using a specific process to put the body and mind in sync. Reducing calories signals the body to repair and rejuvenate, and not worry about stress. In fact, when you're repairing, you actually store less in fat because the body and mind are working together to create health and well-being.

That's the paradigm shift. We start thinking of weight loss as a by-product of healthy living and not something that we desire on its own, and we try to get the body and mind working together so we don't stress the body.

The conscious and unconscious brain

The UdP works with the unconscious brain, which reacts to stress and the inner workings of the organs and the muscles. Let's look at the issues that put the conscious and unconscious brain into conflict, as we transition from content to process.

The hypothalamus was one of the first parts of the brain that developed as humans evolved. It's the area of your brain where you experience worries and fear. The hypothalamus, in concert with numerous other bodily organs and glands, controls your body through hormones, which are slow-acting and long-lasting. With the exception of adrenaline, it takes a while to put a hormone into your circulatory system, and then it takes a while for the effects of that hormone to wear off.

Our hypothalamus basically operates on an unconscious level. We don't think about being hungry, thirsty or tired, or about regulating our body temperature. It just happens: we feel hungry, thirsty, fatigued or cold. When the two systems, our thinking brain and our unconscious system, fight each other, the body will always win.

The first part of our brain developed to survive. The later part developed to control the first part, which built in conflict.

A great example is a job that causes fatigue. If you do 24 hour shift work you struggle to stay awake. You can fight sleep by turning on the TV or drinking coffee. But your body starts grabbing micro naps. You don't even know you fell asleep until you suddenly wake up. That's how people crash cars when they suddenly nod off at the wheel.

The body will win that fight, although it may take a while. That's why you can lose weight while you're thinking about it actively for six to 12 weeks. Coincidentally, that's how long most research studies last, probably because they know people will start gaining the weight back after that time. The study typically lasts for up to 12 weeks and then the body catches up. Then the unconscious brain starts feeling it is in starvation mode, so it pumps out all the hormones necessary to gain the weight back. They are slow-acting, so if we don't directly control them, we're set to fail.

Why "eat less, move more" doesn't work

The subconscious mind and the body work together. Their goal is to prolong life, and to do that they have to make your body as stress-free as possible.

That's part of the reason the resting metabolic rate goes down hours after you've finished exercising. When you are actually exercising, you're using a lot of calories. The only way your body can make up the calories you expend for exercise is to use fewer when you're resting (Hopkins, et al, 2014). That means you relax more and sleep more, and all that time you're not burning or reducing your calories.

For many years, people have been telling us to reduce calories and exercise more to lose weight. The studies don't support that, so we have to look at weight loss differently (Lucan & DiNicolantonio, 2015). We need to shift our emphasis from content to process: not *what to do* but really *why we do it*, and if it makes sense to do it. The hypothalamus is responsible for feelings of hunger. Once the stomach sends the signal to the hypothalamus that it's time to eat, the hypothalamus releases the hormones necessary to make us hungry.

The hormone tells your brain, "I'm hungry," so you start eating. Unfortunately, it takes a long time for that hunger signal to wear off, and you can continue eating even after you are no longer hungry. You use your conscious brain to control what you eat, but when your hypothalamus is in conflict with the conscious brain, it will override it.

The secret fat connection

A recent study looked at the participants of the popular show *The Biggest Loser* five years after the first season (Fothergill, et al, 2014). Of the original 16 contestants, only one had not gained all or most of the weight back. That's significant. These people worked hard for six months, exercising and dieting, and reached the weight they wanted. They were very motivated. Yet all but one of them gained the weight back. Half of them maintained only about a 10% weight loss and gained 90% of the weight back.

Weight is just a data point, but it can show us how well we are controlling stress.

Why would they gain the weight back? It's still speculation but through interviewing the Biggest Loser contestants, it seems that stress had sabotaged their weight loss. It appears that their bodies felt constantly under stress, and this changed their metabolic resting rates (Aamodt, 2016). Now they required fewer calories to maintain their weight than before they had dieted. And they had given up 500 calories a day! So you can see that by eating the same foods as before, in just a year they could gain back 56 pounds while still dieting.

One of the ways to reduce stress is with a paradigm shift where we don't focus on the number on the scale. We focus on healthy activity. We don't set a target because we don't know our ideal body weight. We know that if we reduce stress, the weight will go down because the body doesn't need this excessive fat to save itself. In fact, fat in your body is your ideal food source because it has already been processed. All the impurities have been taken out.

For instance, researchers estimate our brain consumes 20% of the energy in your body. If it doesn't have glucose, which is the sugar in your blood that comes from food, it converts energy directly from your fat and it works almost as well as the glucose. That's how good it is.

The other way to reduce weight is to try to let the body know through your conscious thoughts that you're not going to starve. You can do that through one of the eight principles of the UdP, which is to eat when you're hungry. If you're hungry your body thinks there may not be food, otherwise you would have eaten. In the olden days you grazed for something edible. You would take advantage of finding food because there was less food around than your body required.

In western cultures today it's the opposite problem. Because food is readily available, overeating and weight gain become the issue, not starvation. Marketing and pop culture encourage us to fixate on weight, not wellness. So the UdP helps you make a shift to looking at weight loss not as a goal in itself, but as a by-product of health.

Your weight is a number, and it can go up and down. If you engage in healthy behaviors and you're above your ideal weight, your weight will start going down as you remove stress. In the next chapter, *The 8 Principles of UdP Wellness™*, we'll show you a framework for healthy habits that are sustainable and give you the positive results you want.

CHAPTER 3

8 Principles of UdP Wellness

The Ultimate diet Process (UdP) is designed around eight principles of wellness:

1. **Sustainability**
2. **Eat when you're hungry**
3. **Eat mindfully**
4. **Respect the Triple R day**
5. **Journal every day**
6. **The buddy system**
7. **Find a mentor**
8. **Exercise**

Although they are listed as single principles, they combine to make up the UdP. If you skip one principle, you might be successful for a while, but you will undoubtedly fail in the long run. Let's briefly look at each principle and then see how they work together. We'll examine each one in detail in Part 2 of the book.

The 8 Principles of UdP Wellness

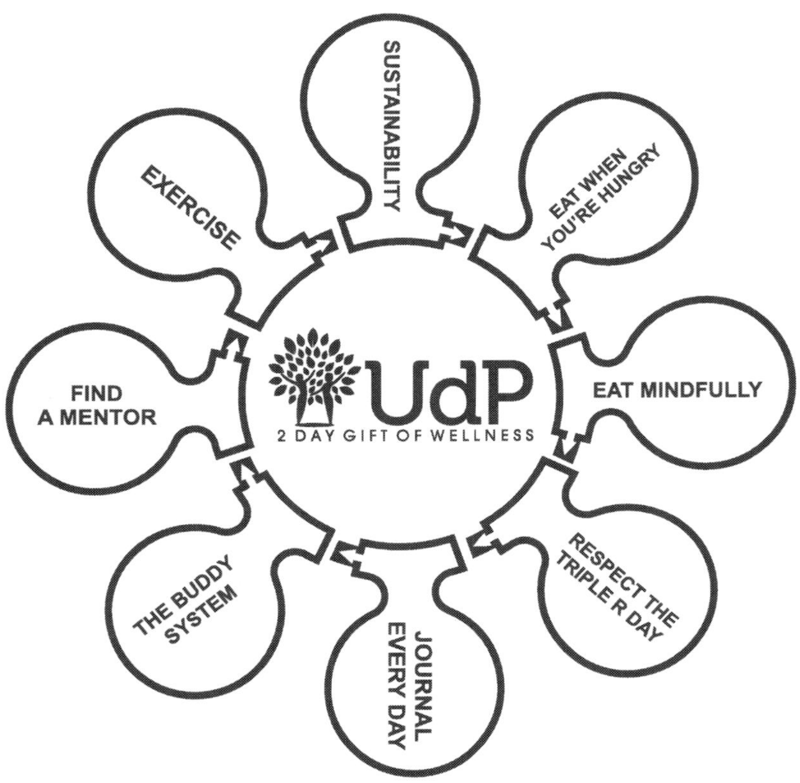

Get a free color chart that you can download here:
www.2dayGift.com/gifts

If you remember the musings from the introduction, we discussed the idea of sticking to the plan. The home builder, who failed at building three houses, decides to modify the plan for his 4th house. His reasoning is clear. He is an experienced homebuilder. After all, he built three houses before.

Of course it's obvious to anyone that his experience is not worth much because all his prior homebuilding projects have failed. In fact his experience is counterproductive and eventually leads to the 4th house collapsing.

So too with dieting. If you are reading this book, I'd wager you have dieted before and might consider yourself somewhat of an expert, despite the fact that your previous diets were not successful in the long run. Repeating things in the same manner and expecting different results is what Einstein called crazy. So commit to following these principles without deviation for the next three months. After that, I know the UdP will be a life process that you will continue forever.

I told my husband that I am doing this [UdP] forever, so he'd better get used to it. – Christie Z

Now that you agree to follow the plan, let me begin to unfold the UdP for you. The first principle is sustainability. The reason it is first is because without the ability to work forever, you don't get off the diet merry-go-round and you may be tempted by the next fad diet. And you now know how that will end, with at least an added 5 pounds.

Sustainability

Sustainability means staying power. The one thing all diets have in common is that they are unsustainable. If they are unsustainable they will fail. The diet industry knows that fact and counts on you forgetting it.

How can you tell if something is sustainable? Ask yourself if you could do this activity forever. For example, if your goal is to exercise for one hour every day, ask yourself honestly if you can do that for the rest of your life. If it's unlikely, then the goal is not sustainable. As you will see in the chapter on sustainability, if it's not sustainable, by definition it will fail.

Because of the critical nature of *sustainability*, every other principle will ask that same question. The answer has to be "yes", or you will have to redesign your question to make it "yes". One way the UdP is sustainable is that you eat when you're hungry.

Eat when you're hungry

Dieting is stressful. When you are hungry, your brain, in concert with your body, sends signals to eat. The brain may override the body's desire to eat by ignoring the request to hunt, gather, cook or eat. The unconscious brain doesn't understand why the food is not there, and thinks there is a food drought.

I don't feel hungry and feel accomplished and proud of myself. I love it [UdP]. – Karen D

The body reacts by becoming ultra-efficient at calorie retention. That means the body learns how to make *fat out of air*. Not literally of course, but it lowers your resting metabolism (the calories your body burns doing nothing). By using the UdP principles, the body understands that not eating is for repairing the body, so it does not go into hyper mode. It uses the rest period for repair and rejuvenation. How does the body know that? Because you eat when you're hungry. Chapter 5 goes deeply into how you do that. But eating when you're hungry is just the beginning. You have to eat mindfully.

It's also interesting to know that the brain requires 20% -25% of our energy consumption, which is about 400 to 600 calories a day. On your Triple R day, almost all your calories are going to power the brain. Maybe that's why most of us feel so creative on a Triple R day.

Eat mindfully

Eating mindfully means thinking about what your brain decides to put into your mouth. To a large degree, the body doesn't care. After all, protein is protein. But you need to pay attention to what you eat. You have to recognize when you are truly hungry, and then decide if you'll have an apple, or an apple tart.

To a large degree, eating mindfully is about nutrition, but not in the typical way. Because the UdP is not prescriptive in what you eat (content), you eat what you enjoy. Eating what you enjoy is about sustainability, which is principle one. But there are rules you can follow that most nutritionists believe will help you feed your body high quality food. In a later part of this book, Debra Thomas, an Integrative Nutrition Health Coach (INHC) shares some insights from her new book on bio-individuality, along with tips for nutritious foods to eat. Bio-individuality is just a fancy way to say our bodies react to foods differently.

You might be wondering how to tell which foods are good for your individual biology. The principle, *journaling every day*, is the primary tool for figuring out that very thing. But first, I must talk about respecting the Triple R day.

Respect the Triple R day – the 2 day gift of wellness

The Triple R day is a day you choose, twice a week, where you reduce, relax, and rejuvenate: the Triple R. All principles are important, but, like sustainability, this principle becomes a focus of the UdP for a couple of reasons.

The first R, **Reduce** speaks to reducing calories to 600 a day, two days a week. You do not reduce calories to lose weight, but to allow your body to repair and rejuvenate. Your body can only repair when you are resting. Resting includes your digestive system. Digesting food uses a lot of energy and is a major focus of the body when you eat (Rohner-Jeanrenaud & Noquerias, 2015). Relaxing at this time is important because if you don't relax, the reduction in calories causes stress, making us hungry and causing the body to go into hyper mode. One rule for the *"relax"* of the Triple R day is: do not intentionally exercise.

Reducing calories twice a week is a type of *intermittent fasting*. Fasting is when you don't eat any food, but with the UdP, you are eating enough to keep the brain going. Anton and Leeuwengurgh in a 2013 meta-analysis of the research said that intermittent fasting is the only known, non-genetic method to increase human lifespan. Yes, I'm talking about living longer. You can see why respecting the Triple R day is so important, and it has nothing to do with weight loss, although that will probably happen as a by-product.

The second R is **Relax**. Relaxing is vitally important for the Triple R. Without relaxing, you have a "calorie reduction only" day, which is unsustainable. "Relax" means doing what you want, procrastinating about stressful events, and taking a day for yourself. The combination of reducing calories and relaxing positively influences our mental attitudes (Mousavi, Rezaei, & Bagnhi, 2014 & Waldo, 2015). Finally, we don't intentionally exercise on a Triple R day, and "relax" is the reason why. Reduce is the engine that drives the Triple R day, and Relax is the catalyst for Rejuvenate, which is the third R.

Rejuvenate is the natural side-effect of the first two Rs. When you reduce stress, relax, and give your digestive system time to recover (reduce), your body understands that this time of rest is for repairing itself. There are studies suggesting that during a fast, the body insulates itself from cancer and actually uses stem cells to completely repair damaged and irreparable cells (Mousavi, Rezaei, Bagnhi, 2014 & Waldo, 2015).

Where do you get the rest of the calories to keep you going? Your body gets it from your stored fat. I'll talk more about this in chapter 7. Before you give up because of the 600 calories, remember it's only two days a week. The rest of the week you eat what you enjoy without counting calories. And besides, you'll have a buddy to help you.

The buddy system

Another feature of sustainability is the buddy system. You can change any habit or craving more successfully when you work with other people (Jackson, Steptoe, & Wardle, 2015; Kluever Romo & Dailey, 2014). The UdP encourages you to go through the process with a partner, friend, co-worker, or family member. You can have different goals, food preferences, work schedules, and ideas about what to eat. This is because the UdP is not content driven. Beyond offering general nutrition advice, I don't even talk about what you should eat. You eat what you enjoy.

Very happy to be experiencing this program with my wife, as it allows us to support each other. Very pleased to see an overall weight loss. – Dave

---

My clients with UdP buddies really encourage each other. They know the lingo. When they say I'm on a Triple R day (or pirate day as Cheri and Pam say, arrr, arrr, arrr), they instantly know what that means. Or if someone expresses frustration about their weight fluctuating, their partner can remind them that weight is just a data point and health is the goal.

Participants who live together create routines for their Triple R days, simultaneously or separately, depending on their weekly or long-term schedules. Even if your romantic partner doesn't initially join, he or she will begin to notice the changes you're experiencing, and probably decide to start the UdP. Your partner will already know the terms. Plus you will now automatically be a mentor, the 7th principle.

Mentor

A mentor is different from a coach or a buddy. Because the UdP is a new process, very few people have gone through it. A coach is helpful, but someone who has not *successfully* completed the process will be mainly a cheerleader (Stelter, 2015). A mentor is a cheerleader, confidant, knowledge provider, and contact when issues arise.

All the UdP mentors at www.2dayGift.com/Mentoring have completed the program and excelled at understanding and putting the principles to work in their lives. They are committed to the UdP lifestyle and to helping as many people as they can. There will be more information in chapter 9, but for now be assured that I will be helping you along the way.

Exercise

The final principle is the one most people associate with weight loss - exercise. I will discuss in detail how exercise is vital to your health and wellbeing. But first I'd like to detangle exercise and weight loss.

One of the tenets of the UdP is to do healthy activities that have weight loss as a by-product. Exercise is the best example. The benefits of exercise in losing weight are mixed. I'll explain how important exercise is - in and of itself. For instance, research suggests if you have to choose weight loss or exercise, choose exercise. Even when obesity is a factor for future health issues, the first priority is exercise (Bouchonville, 2014). Wouldn't it be great if there was a process that had exercise as a principle and weight loss as a by-product?

Now you are beginning to understand the paradigm shift from concentrating on weight loss, which is almost always a fool's errand. Change your life, change your weight. It can be effortless if you concentrate on the correct activities and realize that the scale is only a device to give you an interesting data point on your health and wellness journey.

In Part 2, I will explore each principle in depth and explain the nuts and bolts of actually experiencing this amazing process.

PART 2

Putting the UdP Principles into Action

CHAPTER 4

Sustainability

The reason most diets fail is because they are not sustainable.

Nothing to Worry About

I have to stop that,
It's unsustainable!
That used to worry me a lot.

Then I got a dictionary,
Which stated,
"If it's unsustainable it will stop."

(Ballet in a Coal Mine)

That is precisely what happens to any fad diet, you stop it. There are a variety of reasons to stop a typical fad diet. You decide you don't want to be ruled by points. You don't want to eat just one kind of food. You don't want to buy packaged food and have it shipped to you. You can't eat just meat, just vegetables, or just fruits. Or the rules of the diet are too complicated.

But probably the biggest reason diets fail is because your body, being an open system, adapts to whatever outside influence you experience. In medical terms your body is very accomplished at adapting its metabolism to maintain a set weight. Yes, you can force the body to shed pounds by restricting calories or certain food types, but eventually the body will win.

Research (Fothergill, et al) from 2016 on the first season of the hit show *The Biggest Loser* revealed the latest example of the body's ability to adapt. Six years after spending eight months losing more than 100 pounds each, all but one of the original contestants had gained some of their weight back. The researcher concluded that most of the contestants had "regained a substantial amount of their lost weight in the six years following the competition." They went on to say they consider that quite successful compared to other types of lifestyle interventions. Really? Regaining a substantial amount of weight was considered quite successful?

Weight is a data point with UdP. But weight is also an indicator of your overall stress. Putting back nearly all of your original weight would not be considered a success.

With the UdP, that would not be a success. Although we look at weight as a data point, I expect the weight loss to be permanent once the lifestyle change is made. The researchers in *The Biggest Loser* study attributed the yo-yo effect to metabolic adaption.

It turns out that each of the contestants studied had lowered their resting metabolic rates by an average of 500 calories a day. Yes, a day! That's a significant amount. To put it another way, a person of the same age, gender, and weight could eat a pound of butter a week more than the contestants and not gain weight.

This decreased resting metabolic rate occurs whether the subjects were thin or obese (Rosenbaum, et al., 2008). The researchers concluded that this decline in the amount of energy expended favored weight regain. It seems like the researchers are discovering that permanent weight loss is very unlikely with the weight loss programs available.

These studies are good examples of how the body adapts to stress or crises. But the studies did admit that there is a lot going on, and trying to pin weight regain on rapid weight loss would be a stretch. Maybe the problem is there was no follow-on counseling for these contestants.

Pekkarinen, Kaukua and Mustajoki (2015) looked at that very question. After a group of subjects in a weight loss program completed their program, they divided the subjects into two groups. Each group was equal in terms of weight loss, gender, and age. One group received monthly coaching and the other received no coaching. At the end of a year, the researcher found both groups regained the same amount, regardless of coaching. The study is interesting on two accounts. First, coaching by itself didn't appear to help, and second, weight regain was assumed to occur within a year. So coaching or therapy did not slow down or prevent the weight regain

These studies demonstrate what we already know, that it is almost impossible to lose a significant amount of weight and keep it off with conventional dieting. Karen's story discusses her experiences before UdP, and after.

Karen's story

After over 20 years of failed weight loss efforts, and thousands (literally) of miles walked without significant impact to my weight, I jumped at the chance to be involved with this process. As a two-time cancer survivor, and understanding the positive health impacts of intermittent fasting, the process sounded right to me intuitively.

Before I heard the details (I signed up before I knew), the scariest element was the 600 calorie days. I thought it would be impossible. So before I started the program I tried eating only 600 calories and found it wasn't as hard as I anticipated. The beauty of this process is that it gets easier every single time you do it, almost like a game where you keep trying different things to reach your goal.

The hardest part was disengaging from the social aspect of eating with my family. But there was a bright side to this as well. My family learned that Triple R days were days they were responsible for their own meals (I have two grown children and a husband). This was actually another bonus to the program as I felt I had the "ok" to not be responsible for everyone else's food, something that made me look forward to the "Triple R" days.

The most interesting part of the process and one of the things that makes it so successful is that to reach your 600 calorie goal, you must diminish your intake of processed carbohydrates (they eat up calories crazily fast). You start to make better choices for meals and learn how to cut back calories. When you practice this 2X per week you get better and better at it.

As you plan these days you become aware of the calories you are eating regularly (scary) and realize quickly why you haven't been losing weight. For instance, one day I had 60 calories left and thought I could have about a cup of cashews (I know, DUH), but when I checked the calorie count I quickly realized a large handful of nuts added up to about 10 X what I thought the calorie count was. I was shocked!

As the weeks progressed I became more aware of what I was eating, made better choices (without thinking about it) and ate less as I believe my appetite changed and it took significantly less to fill me up. Miraculously, I changed from a person who lived to eat, to one who eats to live.

I can't emphasize enough that this wasn't based on personal effort from me but happened as a by-product of being engaged in the system. One of the struggles I had, and continue to have, is the relaxation and reflection piece, and sometimes journaling. But I am in a continuous improvement mode. This process even put a stop to my stress eating!

Other positive changes included a reduction in my IBS symptoms, a lack of desire to eat pasta, and better sleep. I now feel in control and know that I will reach my health goals having lost 15 pounds (including while on vacation.) I commit to using this process for the rest of my life. UdP has changed my life in a very positive way. I hope it has the same impact on yours.

Karen's story proves the process is sustainable, but why, exactly? Perhaps a wider view of what's going on is in order. If we look at the body as an open system we can begin to understand. A closed system is like your car. You put gas in and it can go a certain distance. That distance can vary based on how you drive, but the car doesn't make more gas as it approaches empty. The only way the car can go further is by slowing down and reducing drag. The system is closed.

Our body, on the other hand, is an open system. We put energy (calories) in all the time. In the western world we have many more calories available than we could ever use, so the body has three basic options: 1) convert and use the calories as energy 2) eliminate the calories through waste, or 3) store the calories as fat.

The external environment also affects the body's decision. Is food readily available? What physical demands need to be met, such as exercise? Is the body fighting a disease or injury?

The Body's Reaction to Stress

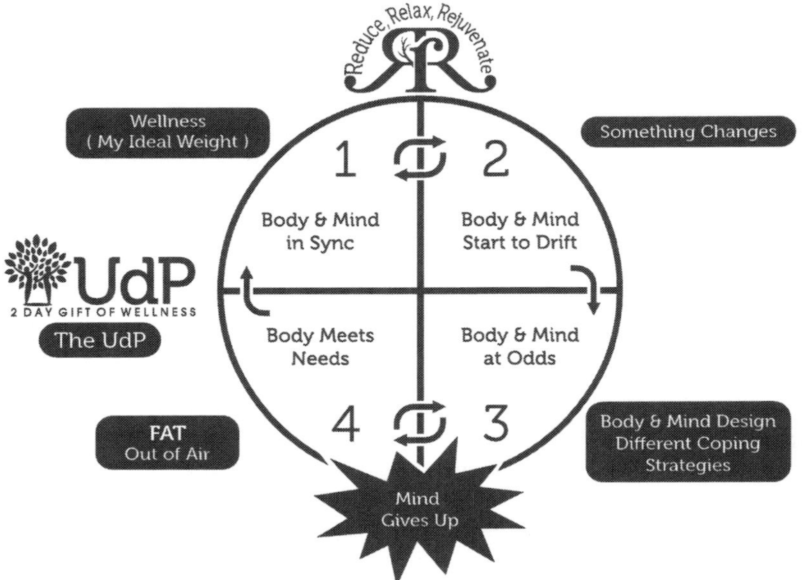

Get a free color chart that you can download here:
www.2dayGift.com/gifts

This model of the body's reaction to stress represents the body as an open system. In an ideal world we start out at our ideal weight and stay there. This is quadrant 1. Quadrant 1 is where we want to return if we are not at our ideal weight. But we will start there to explain the model. If nothing ever changed, we could always stay in quadrant 1, but our body is not a closed system and something always changes. If the change is significant, our conscious mind and our body's weight management system start to drift.

This leads us into quadrant 2, where the body and mind begin to lose sync. If we have a tool like the Triple R day, we can re-sync our mind and body. If not, then the body continues to drift and we gain or regain weight as a result of the body under stress.

In quadrant 3 the mind and body become at odds. The mind might begin to force our body to lose weight by excessive exercise, severe calorie reduction, or a change in diet. The body, meanwhile, still wants to add fat, and this desire only increases when the mind tries to override the body's evolutionary conditioning. This fighting continues until the mind gives up. The body is not wired to give up. It waits until the mind gives up.

In quadrant 4, the body becomes a fat-making machine to get back to the set point it had before all this started. When the stress in quadrants 2 and 3 is high, the body will add a few pounds to fight the next battle with the brain.

The Triple R day is the star, but the other principles of sustainability, eating when hungry, eating mindfully, journaling every day, using your buddy and mentor, and exercising, complete the wellness toolbox.

The body then sets a new point of the weight it wants to maintain. We are not at an ideal weight, but the body figures it's close enough and so goes back to a new quadrant 1, holding on to its new ideal weight. But the mind thinks the weight is too much, so it is out of sync. Being out of sync causes the yo-yo effect and eventually increased weight, until the mind gives up completely at some point.

The UdP was designed to counter this and put us back into a true quadrant 1 where we are at our ideal weight, and body and mind are in sync. This point is called wellness. The UdP can be the positive change agent to drive the body and mind back together, and the Triple R day is the tool to continue this synchronization.

Your goal, then, is to keep yourself in the top half of the model. First, use the UdP to break old habits of dieting and re-dieting where you lose and regain the same pounds, plus a few more. Once you use the UdP to get into quadrant 1, the process becomes sustainable because you proactively use your Triple R days every week to keep the mind and body in sync. But when a significant, unplanned event occurs, you refocus and intensify the Triple R day tools to fight the body's natural tendency to add weight due to stress or change. The additional tools of eating mindfully, journaling, exercising and using your buddy and mentor cement you firmly in the top half of the model, where you live a well-deserved, healthy life.

As you read the remainder of this book, come back to this model and see how the UdP is designed to be sustainable. That trait alone makes this the antidote to the common diet. The simplicity ensures it can be a permanent lifestyle change. The reducing and relaxing parts of the Triple R facilitate the repair and rejuvenation aspects of the UdP. This decreases the likelihood of a significant life change negatively affecting your wellbeing. But you have to follow the plan. One of the most important parts of the process that supports sustainability is the concept of *eating when you are hungry*, the subject of the next chapter.

CHAPTER 5

Eat when you're hungry

When I mentor my UdP folks, I sometimes hear them proclaim, "I feel hungry!" There is a difference between feeling hungry and being hungry. Feeling is an emotion that is not always based on facts. Many things influence feelings, such as daily social activities. If you normally eat when everyone else is eating, you'll want to eat too. So you begin to feel hungry, even if you personally don't need to eat at that time.

How to tell when you're hungry

An important part of the Triple R day is learning to distinguish the feeling of hunger with the physical act of being hungry. It's important every day to know the difference so you can stop eating when your body doesn't need food.

When you reduce to 600 calories, there is a good chance that you will be hungry at some point. That's natural, and when you are hungry you should eat - a primary rule: eat when you are hungry. But mostly, in the beginning at least, "feeling" hungry doesn't mean actual physical hunger.

Triple R days are perfect for discovering the differences. Your day will be distinct from normal days because you plan them better. You start the day by meditating and getting in touch with yourself. You commit to making this day about your body, mind and soul. You commit to being happy, to laughing and enjoying the day as it unfolds, whether you are at work or have a day off. You plan everything you will eat that day, including the time, quality and quantity of your food to maximize the 600 calories.

There is a difference between "feeling" hungry and "being" hungry.

When the day begins, and you start to feel hungry, you should take a quick inventory of the moment. Are you feeling hungry because someone is cooking, or brought in a box of donuts? Is it an eating habit, such as your lunch break, or a snack you always eat at this time? You will get to know what cues are coming from your body, and not from your mind.

If you conclude you are hungry, then eat - period. If you think you are only feeling hungry, don't eat. Distract yourself by taking a walk. Let your mind wander to questions of what makes you happy or what you can do to improve your wellness. At the end of the walk, check in with yourself to see if you are still hungry. Probably not.

By your 4th Triple R day (in 2 weeks) you will have experienced a few good Triple R days, which are days when you weren't hungry at all. Your meals were perfectly planned. Either you grazed all day or you managed the timing perfectly.

Breakfast has been touted as the most important meal of the day. Studies don't back that up. What I often hear is that if you don't eat breakfast, you will be really hungry later. Eating breakfast when you're not hungry is the most common error of the "eat when you're hungry rule." I don't normally eat until after noon. The corollary to eat when you are hungry is *don't* eat when you are *not* hungry.

I have two favorite studies about when to eat. The first one is a wild goose story and the second is a human study. Ho, Wu, Chen and Yang studied the effects of feeding time and time-restricted feeding on the fattening traits of very young white Roman geese. This is a backhanded way of looking at the issue of when to eat. The goal was not to make the geese lose weight, but to gain weight. The study showed conclusively that if fattening up is your goal, the best time to begin feeding geese a high calorie diet is in the morning.

The feeding efficiency (how little food to develop the most fat – belly fat actually) was in the morning. Now think of all the kids being fed cereal, French toast, or donuts first thing in the morning. If you're hungry in the morning, eat high protein, low carb – good ole eggs and bacon. All calories are not equal. The increase in obesity is strongly related to increase in carbohydrates. (Riera-Crichton & Tefft, 2014).

Breakfast is not the most important meal of the day. Eating the first meal when you are hungry is more important.

In the second study, a human study, Chowdhury, et al (2016) found that skipping breakfast did not increase appetite at lunch time. In fact, the researchers found that the subjects did not eat more at lunch, and even after lunch their appetites did not increase. Researchers expected the appetite-stimulating hormone – acylated ghrelin to increase because of the extended morning fast. They were disappointed to see that the hormone actually went down. So, eat when you are hungry, not when history or society tells you to.

Other rules:

Drink when you're thirsty.
Sleep when you're tired.

Simple.

As a rule, I know that I'm not hungry until around noon. So, if I feel hungry at 8 am, I know it is probably a feeling and not hunger. I delay eating, but check back with my body after a distraction. At noon I check in with my body and see if I'm hungry. If I am, I stop what I am doing and fix my meal. If not, I make a mental note to check back in 45 minutes or so.

I don't want to miss or ignore my hunger hints because I never want to be ravenous. Being famished is your body's way of telling you it is very hungry and under stress. We never want our body under stress from lack of calories. Remember, the goal on Triple R days (the 2 day gift of wellness) is to allow your body to repair itself. The body does not repair under stress, it consolidates and turns its attention to storing energy (body fat), which is a primary survival mechanism.

Your tools on Triple R days are your UdP buddy, your mentor, and your journal. Use all three tools to discover for yourself when you are feeling hungry or when you are hungry.

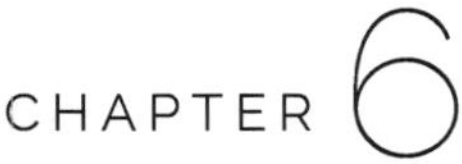

Eat mindfully & nutritionally

Whenever people tell me they eat healthy food but still can't lose weight, I ask them if they practice eating mindfully. Most people stare back at me blankly or ask me what on earth I'm talking about.

Today, we often eat on the go, grabbing a fast bite at our desk, in our cars, and even walking in the street. We may be eating for quick sustenance, but when we wolf down food under stress, our bodies don't absorb the nutrients. That's why we often feel tired and our brains don't function optimally.

A wealth of scientific data shows that eating quickly, not chewing thoroughly, and not paying attention to what and how much we eat can result in substantial overeating. Even healthy foods can cause weight gain if we eat too much of them.

What Did I Eat?

A hidden bonus section on nutrition

By Debra Thomas, Integrative Nutrition Health Coach (INHC)

When we notice we are bloated, gassy, tired, aching, have a headache, itching, lethargic, or have digestive issues, constipation, or diarrhea, one of the first questions we should ask ourselves is **"what did I eat?"** It always comes back to food. The Institute for Integrative Nutrition®, coined the phrase *bio-individuality*™ which simply means everyone's body reacts to food differently.

Food provides the body with the energy needed to function throughout the day. If we are not energized by what we eat, that food can no longer be considered a good food, no matter how healthy and organic it is. We might have a micro-allergy.

Unfriend stress & anyone that causes you stress.

Everyone is familiar with food allergies. But the typical food allergy, such as celiac disease, which is a life threatening reaction to gluten, is not the most common allergy. Micro-allergies are small, but noticeable negative reactions to food. Some people also call these reactions *food intolerances.* These reactions are not life-threatening, but they do cause stress to our digestive system and must be identified and left out of our daily food intake.

The best way to find out what foods are making you sick is to journal. Journaling should become a part of your life, forever. Journaling is one of the most important principles of the Ultimate diet Process (UdP). You journal what you are thinking, eating, doing, and how you feel each time. You put your deepest, most private thoughts, and your goals and accomplishments, in your journal. You share only what you want to. If you don't want to share something, keep it private.

Fasting is important to acquiring a healthy body and lifestyle. Fasting does not mean you do not eat or you only drink liquids for a certain amount of time. Fasting is getting away from stress. Let your body rejuvenate, relax and rest. Ideally, fast 2 days a week, two or three days apart, by cutting your calorie intake to around 600 calories on those days to help your body regenerate. This, of course, is the Triple R day of the UdP. As Dr. Christensen writes, it is your *2 day gift of wellness.*

Juicing and drinking organic bone broth are wonderful ways to help your body heal at a cellular level. This is also the time you meditate, pray, focus on your spirituality, and ponder questions that make you think on a different level. Fasting will also help you fine tune your concentration, your clarity, and your overall health. Above all, reduce stress. Stress, whether mental or physical, is not your friend. "Unfriend stress!"

If you are having troubles identifying your micro-allergies, use another important principle of the UdP - hire a coach. I recommend a certified coach who understands and uses a wide variety of dietary and nutritional theories. It's important that he or she understand the UdP and can apply the 8 principles. The synergy of the UdP and a nutrition coach can integrate both nutrition and wellness to support your overall health.

Debra Thomas is a Life Path Health Coach. Find out more here: **www.LifePathHealthCoach.com**

Look for hidden sources of micro-allergies or food intolerances

These 7 triggers cause about 90% of food allergies or intolerances.

1. Peanuts
2. Fish & shellfish
3. Eggs
4. Soy
5. Wheat
6. Tree nuts such as walnuts, pecans and almonds
7. Milk and dairy products such as cheese, yogurt and ice cream

You may think you are avoiding eggs or cheese by not eating a cheese omelet for breakfast, but each of these foods can be hidden in a surprising variety of packaged and processed foods. For example, did you know that barbecue sauces made with Worcestershire sauce may contain anchovies? Milk, eggs, and soy are used in a vast number of packaged foods, everything from baked goods to salad dressings, sauces, mashed potatoes, and even chewing gum.

Again, this is where journaling can help you. By recording what you eat every day, you'll note any reactions, and trace them back to your recent meals. If you suspect you have an intolerance to any food, try eliminating that food for a few days and see if your symptoms subside. Don't try to eliminate several foods at once, or you won't know what caused your symptoms. Test one food at a time.

Food allergies or intolerances can be difficult to diagnose on your own. It's a good idea to consult your doctor or a qualified nutritionist for testing, to help you figure out what's causing your food reactions. Once you know which foods you react to, your health will improve as your body won't have to struggle to digest those foods. You may find it easier to lose weight if that's your goal.

Top nutritious foods to fill up on

Here is a handy list of nutritious foods for your Triple R days, and for every day! But remember, you must enjoy the food you eat. Don't force yourself to eat anything you find distasteful. This process is about sustainability. If you can't see yourself eating something the next year or even the next week, don't eat it. If you like meat or enjoy a protein based diet, then eat that. But if you want to expand your palate, these are good rules to follow.

A simple rule of thumb is to "eat the rainbow." Eat a variety of fresh fruits and vegetables every day – the darker the color, the more vitamins and minerals you get. Choose organic and non-GMO whenever possible, to avoid pesticides and preservatives that can wreak havoc with your weight, and even worse, undermine your health.

- **Fresh leafy greens:** A salad a day keeps the doctor away. The darker the greens, the more vitamins and minerals.
- **Cruciferous vegetables:** Brussel sprouts, broccoli, cauliflower, kale, cabbage and many more of these nutritious vegetables are known to decrease the risk of cancer and other diseases.
- **Fresh fruit:** All berries are excellent and low in fat. The darker the fruit, the more nutrients it contains, so look for red and purple fruits such as grapes, plums, and watermelon. Any fruit the size of your palm, such as an apple, orange, or peach makes a tasty snack that is great for you.
- **Peas, beans and lentils:** With over 20 different species of legumes varying in shape, texture, color, and taste, legumes make a perfect all-season food, from hearty chili in winter to a fresh bean salad at a summer BBQ. They are nutritious, inexpensive and versatile. Legumes are an excellent low fat meat alternative, providing protein, fiber, B vitamins and iron.
- **Sprouted grains and micro greens:** From alfalfa to broc-

coli, and oats to buckwheat, sprouts and micro greens (baby plants in their prime) are living foods. They are high in proteins and among the most complete and nutritional foods that exist, with the highest concentration of nutrients per calorie of food, so they fill you up and help with weight loss.

- **Healthy oils:** Get your oil from avocados and olives, and avoid corn, canola and vegetable oils which are highly processed.
- **Fish:** If you eat fish, go for the cold water fish such as salmon, sardines, herring, and mackerel, and try to get wild fish, not farmed.
- **Lean organic meat:** If you eat meat, choose organic chicken, turkey or beef to avoid the hormones and antibiotics in conventionally raised animals.
- **All spices**: Spices are wonderful for your health. Add ginger, cayenne pepper, turmeric, cumin, cardamom, and cinnamon to your food for a boost in flavor and health.
- **Raw nuts and seeds:** Choose from a wide variety of nuts and seeds including almonds, walnuts, pumpkin, and sunflower seeds. Be careful of the amounts, as they have healthy fats, but are high in calories. A small handful of nuts are rich and satisfying, and stop hunger pangs.
- **Garlic and onions:** Plants in the allium family such as onions, garlic, scallions, leeks and chives are powerful medicinal plants that have been used for centuries to prevent or cure disease and support a healthy immune system. They add flavour to your meals, with hardly any calories.

Nutrition and eating mindfully are important principles to use every day. Journaling and hiring a mentor are principles to help you discover your micro-allergies and food intolerances. These three principles occupy a special place in the 2 day gift of wellness: The Triple R day.

CHAPTER 7

Triple R day™

Your 2 Day Gift of Wellness

The Triple R day is a simple process, but it's not easy, especially at the beginning. It's simple because you really only do two things: eat responsibly, and relax.

The first thing to keep in mind is to eat when you're hungry. This is especially important on Triple R days, but on regular days as well. The second thing to remember is that this is a long-term, sustainable process. We know that diets make you gain weight, so we don't want to make it a diet.

The main thing is to make the main thing the main thing. – Steven Covey

---

Your goal is to develop healthy habits and activities that have weight loss as a side benefit. We're approaching this as a process where your mind and body come together for healthy living. If you're experiencing stress, your body thinks it's under attack and you can't reach your ideal weight.

You'll be journaling every day to record what you ate, when and why you ate it, and how the food made you feel. Let's look at the three components of the Triple R day.

Part 1: Reduce

Reducing calories is only one part of the Triple R. All diets that promise weight loss reduce calories. Most reduce calories every day. For instance you can go to websites (https://www.bcm.edu/cnrc-apps/caloriesneed.cfm) or apps and figure out how many calories you need to eat to maintain or lose weight. In previous chapters, we have shown that the body has biological set points that it fights to maintain. The body simply becomes more efficient at using the calories you give it. The body also rests without you knowing it by lowering its metabolic rate.

Any reduction in calories must be sustainable for permanent weight loss.

Using a calorie-in-calorie-out (eat less – exercise more) scenario, all you have to do is reduce your calories by 500 a day (or increase your exercise by 500 calories a day) and you'd lose 1 pound a week. In the exercise section, you'll learn what you already know: this scheme never works for a number of reasons (accurate counting of calories, accurate recording of food, sustainability, etc).

You could reduce calories on certain days. These types of diets are alternate- fasting type diets. For instance, you might reduce your intake to be eating nothing, or about 600 calories every other day. If you can keep that up, and don't increase your calorie intake on regular days, you have a decent chance of reducing your weight. But, (and this is a big but), this type of diet does not reset your weight point because your body is always under stress. While you're reducing calories every day, the body is reconfiguring to make up for the reduction. As soon as your mind (willpower) gives up, you'll quickly regain a large portion of the weight you lost. In short, for most people it is not sustainable. Sustainability is a core principle in the UdP. That rules out an alternate-day fasting diet.

A much more sustainable fast is to fast a few times a week (one, two, three or four days). Mathematically, three or four equates to essentially every other day. That really leaves one or two days a week. I chose two days a week. Physiologically, one isn't enough and three is too many. Like the fairy tale Goldilocks, the middle amount was just right. Two days a week is sustainable IF you do it correctly. In our case it's sustainable if you follow the other principles of UdP and the remainder on the Triple R days (Rest and Rejuvenate). Without the two additional R's and the other 7 principles, you are doing a 5:2 style diet that is not sustainable and may not reset your weight point towards your ideal weight.

Fasting the UdP way

Two days a week, separated by at least one day, you reduce your calories to a total of 600, which is approximately 25% of your normal calorie intake. There is no requirement to eat or avoid any specific foods. However, some foods such as proteins and fats, have greater staying power. Those two days are the only days a week that we count calories. I suggest variety and small meals throughout the day, but you can do whatever works for you so you don't get hungry. Some of my clients find the repetition of similar foods (different types of egg dishes, for instance) keeps their hunger under control. Others find a day full of vegetables works great and fits into their organic, non-GMO lifestyle.

This is not a content driven process, so you fill in the details of how you want to eat your 600 calories. There are suggestions and recipes in the back of the book. Christie's story is full of ways to make 600 calories work. The internet is also full of 600 calorie recipes. I like to break my day into a 150 calorie noon meal, a 150 calorie afternoon snack and then a 300 calorie dinner. But you can decide what works for you.

This is where a UdP mentor would really come in handy. Also if you join one of the 2daygift.com mentoring groups, you will get multiple ideas from all the people going through the process with you. That's why I highly encourage you to join one of my groups. Your individual chances of succeeding in the UdP will approach 100%. I find that the closer you follow ALL the principles (especially respecting the Triple R, journaling, UdP buddy, and mentor), the happier you will be with your wellness.

Go to www.2dayGift.com/Mentoring and join a mentoring and buddy group today. You will be happier with your results.

The other days (non-Triple R days) you mindfully eat what you enjoy. You don't keep track of calories or even portion size. You just list what you eat in your daily journal.

Fasting: the best thing you can do for your body

Recall the core concept of UdP; we don't fast 2 days a week to lose weight, *we fast for the health benefits*. Remember your paradigm shift? We do healthy activities that have weight loss as a side effect. Did you know that fasting was a healthy activity?

You've had plenty of hints. Almost all major religions of the world have fasting as a core principle. For instance:

- Buddhism uses fasting during intense meditation retreats.
- Christianity use fasting to develop a closer relationship to God.
- Hinduism has fasting as integral to the religion.
- Islam lists fasting as the forth of the Five Pillars of Islam. Most of us are familiar with the holy month of Ramadan, where fasting is required from sun up to sun down.

We use fasting for its many health benefits. For instance Anton & Leeuwenburgh in 2015 completed a study on the benefits of fasting on life span. During their search of the current state of scientific research they commented that fasting is the only proven, non-genetic intervention that you or I can do to positively increase our life span.

That's a powerful statement. That statement alone makes fasting a "must do" event for long term wellness. Anton & Leeuwenburgh's study looked at oxidative stress. Basically, *oxidative* stress is the difference in the body's ability to detoxify or to repair damage. Oxidative stress is important to reduce because it is thought to be involved in the development of:

- Asperger syndrome
- ADHD
- Cancer
- Parkinson's disease
- Lafora disease
- Alzheimer's disease
- Atherosclerosis
- Heart failure
- Myocardial infarction
- Fragile X syndrome
- Sickle cell disease
- Lichen planus

- Vitiligo
- Autism
- Infection
- Chronic fatigue syndrome
- Depression

How does fasting do this? That's a good question, and one that continues to be studied. The basic theory is that fasting deregulates (turns off) the genes involved in oxidative stress, increasing the body's ability to detoxify and repair cells. When you fast, the brain can actually take stem cells from your body for repair. This helps enhance your cellular control, both in your brain and throughout your body. Instead of duplicating that bad cell or trying to repair one that's beyond repair, it uses another stem cell to make a whole new cell.

Fasting is proven to increase lifespan and fight disease.

Fasting has been shown to increase mental health. A study by *The Journal of Fasting and Health*, stated that people who fast, reported decreases in anxiety, depression, and insomnia. In addition, they reported increased ability to handle social functions (Mousavi et al, 2014).

An important consideration for any weight loss program or process like the UdP is eating disorders. Some fad diets, without intention, might encourage people susceptible to eating disorders to fall back into their bad habits. A very important aspect of intermittent fasting (like we do in UdP) is that it helps control unrestrained eating behaviors (Hoddy, et al, 2015). Intermittent fasting either discourages or helps to positively control:

- Binge eating
- Purgative behavior
- Fear of fatness
- Avoidance of forbidden foods
- Increased body image perceptions.

UdP was designed with eating disorder prevention in mind. That is why we use weight as a data point, not a goal. Setting a goal of a certain weight by a certain time may encourage bad eating behaviors (Ordonez, Schweitzer, Galinsky, & Baserman, 2009). I remember that in high school several wrestlers took laxatives, ran in plastic suits, purged food, and starved themselves to make weigh-in. As soon as these wrestlers had weighed in, they'd binge eat, and try to recover the strength they'd lost doing those harmful behaviors.

The UdP was designed to counter eating disorders caused by dieting.

UdP combats eating disorders by only reducing calories two days a week, and only to 600 calories. On non-Triple R days, there is no counting or restricted food. If you are following the 8 principles you will eat mindfully, journal daily, confide in your UdP buddy group, exercise, eat only when you are hungry, and understand that this is not a get-thin-quick plan. It is designed to teach good eating habits and to be a sustainable way of life. Take that, eating disorders!

Also, reducing to 600 calories decreases your biological stress. This is connected to disease prevention, and both animal and human trials have shown this to be true. In animal trials, they've given TRAMP mice prostate cancer and watched as the cancer grew (Bonorden, et al, 2009). For the mice on intermittent fasting regimes, the onset of cancer was delayed. If the mice developed cancer, the symptoms were slower to appear, which meant a longer lifespan.

Obviously we can't do that with humans, but you can do trials with people who have cancer and see how intermittent fasting affects them. It's been shown that fasting also helps protect against the development of cardiovascular disease or metabolic diseases such as thyroid issues, and helps enhance insulin sensitivity. Fasting is even shown to prolong reproductive functions in people. Studies also show that fasting helps with neuron regeneration, and helps stops neuron degeneration related to Parkinson's and Alzheimer's.

One of the most important reasons to reduce calories is to give your body a pause from digesting. The body harnesses a tremendous amount of energy to transform the food we eat into energy or fat we can use, and this is especially true if you eat junk food (Rohner-Jeanrenaud & Noqueiras, 2015). Just by reducing digestion, your body can spend the energy it needs to repair your cells.

Your body loves using the fat you've already stored, which is especially good if you're overweight. You just have to provide the incentive. Think about it like this. Fat is like your savings account. If you can convince your body that you have too much in your account, the easiest way for it to get energy is to withdraw it right from the "fat savings account."

Part 2: Relax

Relaxing gives your mind and body a break. Without the relaxing component, you're just eating a low calorie diet. I bet you think, "I got this relaxing part down!" My clients say this is the hardest part of the UdP – relaxing. I don't know if it's because of our culture, but the clients grab on to the reducing part like a dog on a bone, but can't work in time to relax.

The reason my clients can reduce is because that is what they are good at. They all have experience dieting and are good at it. They've all lost 100's of pounds over their life time. They also have gained more back over the same period. But the UdP is different in many ways than a diet. One thing we know about low calorie diets is that they are not sustainable (Aamodt, 2016). Studies show that you get tired of restricting calories and after six or eight months you go back to your old ways. To continue the Triple R days for the rest of your life, you need the incentive of relaxation.

Happiness

Happiness has been discussed as a life goal throughout the ages. Aristotle and Plato even had examples of how to increase your happiness. They believed that all human beings have an innate desire to be happy. They felt that happiness is obtainable and teachable. And believe it or not, although it's subjective, happiness is measurable (Sato, et al, 2015). You can see when people report that they're happy but this is strongly influenced by genetics, your emotional state and how you frame your feelings. If you think you are having a bad day, you're having a bad day.

Meditating

Meditating and relaxing help with anxiety, depression and insomnia. It has also been shown to increase your social functions and the way you deal with other people (Mousavi, et al, 2014). When you meditate using the deep Triple R day questions in part 3, you get to know yourself better. This allows you to get rid of activities that are destructive and are causing you pain. The absence of pain is pleasurable, especially if you've been dealing with chronic pain and stress.

Begin each day by making your mind still. Find a quiet spot to stop thinking; stop worrying, stop stressing, stop planning your day, and stop multi-tasking. Pico Lyer, delivering a Ted Talk in 2014 said, "In an age of acceleration, nothing can be more exhilarating than going slow. And in an age of distraction, nothing is as luxurious as paying attention. And in an age of constant movement, nothing is so urgent as sitting still."

If you are having a hard time stilling your mind, you can use a combination of a mantra and breathing. A mantra is a sentence or two that you repeat. For me, I use this simple one, based on the Serenity Prayer by the theologian, Reinhold Niebuhr.

Morning Mantra on Important Matters

Please provide me:
Humility to accept what
I cannot change,

Courage to change what I can,
Wisdom to discern the difference.
Amen (rinse & repeat)

(Ballet in a Coal Mine)

Breathing

A very important part of relaxing is learning to breathe. When you have stilled your mind, start an inhale from the bottom of your diaphragm. As you inhale, imagine a pure white mist entering your body through your nose and mouth. Make this breath slow and very deep. When you feel the need to exhale, slowly let the breath out and imagine all your bad energy and thoughts flowing out of your head. Repeat this for 10 minutes.

It even helps if you have a very quiet bell that will ring at the end of 10 minutes.

Just before your ten minutes are up, you might feel what Max Christensen (no relation) calls skin breathing. Your inhales and exhales are so connected that you don't feel the breathing at all. According to Christensen (2014) this is the beginning of feeling bliss. When you hear the bell, slowly allow your mind to become aware of your surroundings. You should feel calm.

Laughing

Another exercise is called laughing. Yes, just like you can measure happiness, you can change your mood by laughing. But what, you might ask, can you do to laugh? That's where the simple exercise comes in. Find a quiet place and just say Ha, Ha, He, He. Say it over and over again and soon you will be laughing with a big grin on your face. My wife and I did this in a large home improvement store. We got some looks, but we got some laughs too. And we grinned all the way home. I'm grinning right now, just remembering it. By the way, short-hand for laughing in the UdP is H4.

Choose a job you love, and you will never have to work a day in your life. - Confucius

---

Of course it would be easier to relax if you don't have to work. Work is often the big fly in the ointment. You can do one Triple R day on the weekend, but the other day you have to work, so how do you manage that? We'll discuss this a little more in a following section. The most important thing about relaxing at work is to plan for a relatively easy day. Pick the easiest day of your week and make it easier by planning ahead. The best advice I have is to plan your Triple R day early in the week. That way you can reschedule it for later in the week if something unexpected comes up.

Part 3: Rejuvenate

Rejuvenating and repairing are byproducts of reducing and relaxing. Your body repairs automatically but you have to help it along, which is why you don't intentionally exercise on your Triple R days.

You can get unintentional exercise by doing something you enjoy such as going for a walk or a bike ride. But don't plan to speed walk, sprint, or lift heavy weights. If you are going to the gym for something other than a massage, sauna, or stretching yoga, you're not respecting the Triple R day.

Also avoid multitasking on Triple R days. If you're using technology and double-task by checking your email while you work, you're not giving your mind a chance to relax so your body doesn't have a chance to repair. Give yourself a break. Allow your body to rejuvenate by replacing defective cells with stem cells- brand new cells that help you live longer. Your body won't do that if it's under stress.

One more benefit: when you give your body time to repair, you'll find yourself becoming more creative. Relaxing also helps repair your emotions. You feel happier when you're relaxed. One of my clients claimed she became more intuitive. Another said she was so happy when she had her first restful night's sleep at the end of her Triple R day. I began writing this book, editing another, and writing a third. I don't feel stress doing them, I just do them. I pick up my ukulele more often, just for the joy of singing.

After a couple of weeks, you will get the hang of the Triple R day. It's very important that you respect it and everything it requires. The Triple R days are your 2 day gifts of wellness. Soon you will look forward to the cleanse, the "me" time, the stress free days, and the creativity that only a Triple R day can bring. The 2 day gifts are simple, but you still need to plan them carefully, at least at first.

4 Steps to planning a great Triple R day

Now that we've talked about what to do on a Triple R day, let's talk about how to schedule and plan your day so you feel great, and have an enjoyable experience.

Step 1: Schedule your day

On Sunday, look at your journal from the past week and ask yourself: "How did my week go? What will next week look like? Which two days will I pick for Triple R days, making sure to separate them by at least one day?"

Now pick your Triple R days for the coming week, based on what you anticipate will be your most and least stressful days. They may not always be weekends or days off.

For example, if Wednesdays are usually light work days, then schedule your Triple R day for Wednesday. If you know Monday is generally a hectic day because messages tend to pile up from the weekend, don't schedule your Triple R day on Monday.

If Wednesday is your Triple R day, you'll stop eating after dinner on Tuesday, abound 7 or 8 pm. You'll be eating 600 calories on Wednesday and then resume normal eating when you end your Triple R day on Thursday at breakfast or lunch.

Step 2: Plan your food for your Triple R day

Triple R days are really the only days you'll have to plan ahead to have specific foods available. The idea is to graze all day. This allows you to eat mindfully and only when you're hungry.

The day before your Triple R day, make a menu and shop for your food for that day. You get 600 calories, which can be a lot of food or not much, depending on what you select.

We've provided some top foods for nutrition in the nutrition chapter, and some sample 600 calorie menus with recipes in the back of the book to help you.

Step 3: Manage your eating

You don't have to eat three meals and two snacks just because menus are often set up that way. When you eat only when you're hungry, you might have six or eight snacks a day. If you get hungry, eat, and don't let yourself become ravenous. If you get busy or you know you'll be away from the house for a while, bringing a nutritious snack such as a hardboiled egg or an apple with a few nuts can keep you from grabbing fast food that will sabotage your day. If you get too hungry you put your body under stress, and it's harder to relax again. The goal is to control your appetite and not let yourself become famished.

The real secret to the Triple R day is to Schedule, Plan, Manage, and Do! It really is that simple.

Step 4: Do relaxing, fun activities

The day before a Triple R day, organize activities that will help you relax and make you happy, including spending time with family and friends. Plan to get a massage or a manicure. Arrange a golf game or a bike ride. Enjoy activities such as a stroll or a swim, and skip the gym and any strenuous exercise.

Start your day by meditating to clear your mind. I use a generic term, because there are many types and traditions of meditation around the world. All the major religions have a form of meditation, including prayer. The idea is to still your mind and give your problems up to the universe or to God. This decreases your mental stress while increasing your happiness.

Commit to reducing stress and having a happy day. Push anything unpleasant to the next day whenever possible. You want to plan your day, and manage it as it evolves. Part of relaxing is to feel blissful, and to be blissful, you have to laugh.

Another example of planning your day is to attribute good intentions to people you meet. By that I mean, don't assume their intentions are bad. If you get cut off, it was an accident. If someone takes your parking spot, they need to hurry back to take care of a sick wife. It's only for today, but maybe assuming good intentions will carry over to every day.

Remember, you create your Triple R days by relaxing and feeling happy. That's how you go through this process. Practice your Triple R day techniques every day of the week, so you are happy every day. Why be miserable on days you eat what you enjoy, without worrying about calories? You should be deliriously happy those days!

Triple R days in the workplace

On your Triple R day at work, the more you arrange your day in advance, the easier it will be. Showing up with a care-free attitude helps keep you from getting stressed. But what if you have more work than you can possibly do?

If you can't possibly get all the work done, don't stress – it's impossible. But what is possible is to work on important but not urgent work.

Steven Covey in his ground-breaking book *7 Habits of Highly Effective People* suggests this matrix of how to divide work. I use it to decide what I want to work on during my Triple R day.

As you can see from the matrix, quadrant 1 is important and urgent. These are activities you must do. But you really don't have as many of these as you think you do, so go through your tasks carefully – the day before! As you plan your Triple R work day, ask yourself these question, "Is this task urgent? Is this task important?" Any task that is not important and not urgent (quadrant 4) goes to the shredder or may be delegated.

	Urgent	Not Urgent
Important	Crying baby Kitchen fire Some calls 1	2 Exercise Vocation Planning
Not Important	3 Interruptions Distractions Other calls	4 Trivia Busy work Time wasters

The hardest quadrant to control is quadrant 3. In quadrant 3 are unimportant things that are urgent. A ringing phone or text message demands your urgent attention, but probably isn't critical unless you are expecting an important call. Coworkers wanting to vent about the boss, their spouse, and their children appear urgent, but are not important. You need to figure out how to avoid giving these unimportant interruptions any time. Turn off your cell phone. Don't log on to Facebook, Twitter, SnapChat, or whatever is the newest craze. They waste time, but more importantly they will stress you out because you are not doing the important work you need to do.

The only quadrant left is quadrant 2 - important but not urgent. Why would you work on these items if they are not urgent? That's exactly why you work on them during Triple R days. Quadrant 2 activities have long-term payoffs. When you finish important and urgent work, the only other activity you should do is important but not urgent. Your boss or bottom line will appreciate your strategic thinking. Because it's not due tomorrow, there's no stress if you can't complete the important task – it's not even due yet!

The goal, then, is to do things that are important but aren't urgent. These are things that you want to do but don't have a deadline. It could be working on business plans, or organizing your office.

Another fine plan is to procrastinate with purpose. Normally, procrastination is a bad word, but on a Triple R day, it is beneficial to put off stressful tasks. To procrastinate with purpose, schedule your day to work on things that you need to do but you don't have a looming deadline. This could be strategic or career planning. Now, if your Triple R day gets derailed because your boss needs you to handle an urgent project, simply reschedule your Triple R day to later in the week.

The more quadrant 2 issues you manage now, the fewer quadrant 1 issues you will face in the future.

I have one client who plans Tuesday thru Friday as a Triple R day. Like me she doesn't usually eat until noon, so she brings a 150 calorie egg omelet in for lunch. By lunch time, she usually knows how the day will go. If it looks good, she makes the day her Triple R day and only has 4 hours left of work. Pretty smart thinking, and planning the night before for her work days decreases her stress all week long. Several times she has completed both her Triple R days at work. But usually, she plans a weekend day for herself.

CHAPTER 8

Journaling

Christie's story

Christie's story: The mind/body/spirit connection

Before finding the UdP, I was ready to make some changes in my life. I had declared 2016 the year of getting healthy. I had gone to the doctor earlier in the year and had been chastised because I hadn't had any of the routine health checkups in years.

I am not fond of doctors because I feel they throw medications at conditions rather than looking for the cause: reactive medicine practices versus proactive.

I scheduled all the necessary appointments and everything came back clear so I felt like the next piece was to address my diet. I know which foods are healthy but still had issues losing weight.

When the opportunity to participate in the UdP program was presented, I felt like it made sense. There were no gimmicks.

I loved that the "Triple R" days were focused not just on reducing calories but reducing stress as well. For me, it addressed the "mind, body, spirit" connection. Those days gave me an opportunity to take time out for myself, which I rarely do.

They gave me an opportunity to reset. I started to listen to my body and what it needed rather than stuffing it with food. In daily journaling, I was able to see how much I was eating and when. Then I was able to figure out why. Was I hungry, tired, bored, stressed?

I hadn't realized how much I was eating. Even eating healthy, when you consume too much food, isn't good for you. At the beginning, it was difficult as I adjusted to eating less food on Triple R days.

Again, it went back to listening to my body. I also had a hard time relaxing and putting myself first, putting off things that may cause stress that could wait until the next day.

As the weeks went by and the weight loss continued, it became obvious to me that this was a process I could sustain. The weight has been coming off very slowly but that doesn't bother me. The fact is, it is coming off.

I began to feel more grounded, more at peace.

Each week the number is a little lower than the week before. In the past, this may have bothered me. I wanted immediate gratification. Since this program isn't just about weight loss, I started to measure my success in other ways than just weight loss. I noticed that I was feeling more grounded, more at peace, in spite of the fact that there were some very stressful things happening during the period of testing.

Usually when I was under a lot of stress, I would throw any healthy habits out the window and engage in things that weren't good for me, such as overeating, eating junk or processed food, and drinking too much alcohol.

With the UdP, I overindulged for a couple of days here and there. But each day I could reset, instead of feeling like I had to start again the following Monday, blowing off the rest of the week.

After 3 months on the program, I definitely feel it is sustainable. It has become my way of life. I was also able to participate in this program with my spouse. Although our approach was completely different, I think it helps to have a partner who knows what you are going through. They are familiar with the UdP lingo. We were able to support each other through the process.

Christie's 2 month progress

Christie was chosen because her journaling is so complete. She lost about 5.5 pounds a month, which was typical. Her 1 pound bump in weight in week 6 was because of a vacation, but she was still losing over time.

Pounds lost by Christie

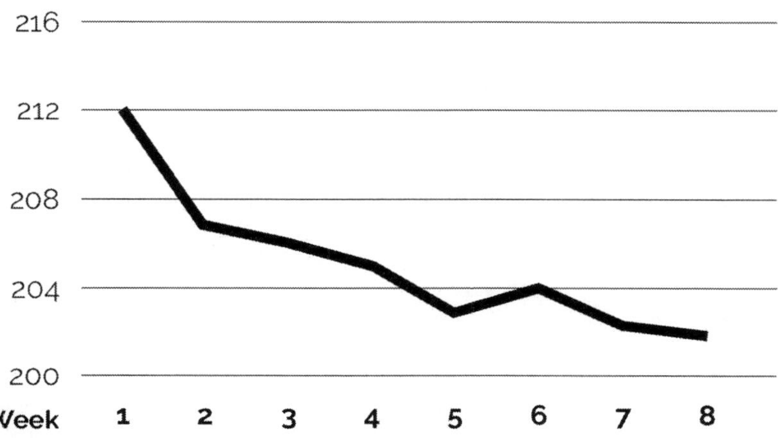

A core principle is to journal every day, even when it is not a Triple R day. Other days are important for discovering micro-allergies, as stated in the nutrition section. Remember, you do not have to be so detailed on regular days, unless it helps you. Here are some important points about journaling:

1. Journal every day. Pick a time in the morning or evening and make it a commitment. If you are participating in a www.2daygift.com mentoring and buddy accountability program, the online journal fills this requirement.

2. Weigh yourself several times a day, if you can. Only record the lowest weight in your journal. Weight varies by what you eat, what activities, what time of day you weigh yourself, etc. By always picking the lowest number you'll be consistent. Weight will fluctuate, but is only an indicator of your wellness at that moment. If you are over your ideal weight (as your body determines, not fashion or conventional standards), as your wellness improves, your weight will trend downwards. Remember you are setting new weight points as you slowly increase wellness without the stress of dieting.

3. Keep track of your sleep. Studies show if you aren't getting more than 6.5 hours, you are compromising your wellness and weight loss. Sleep is vital.

4. Record your physical activities. I recommend a pedometer of some sort (smart watch, smart phone, Fitbit, etc). A pedometer will keep track of your steps. Steps will probably be the only activity you record on Triple R days. Do not go to the gym except for a sauna, massage, or stretching/yoga type activity. When you begin to work out on weeks 2 and beyond, keep track of what you are doing on your non-Triple R days. Remember, exercise and weight loss are not joined at the hip. You can exercise and not lose weight, and you can lose weight without exercising.

5. Hours/Calorie Reduced. These are hours that you lived on 600 calories. For example on Christie's first Triple R day (Tuesday) she finished her last meal at 8pm Monday night. She didn't eat on Wednesday until 9am, so 4+24+9 = 37 hours of fasting on 600 calories. If she does that twice in one week, she has lived 74 hours (37x2) on only 1200 calories (600x2), and didn't get hungry.

6. "Notes" are where you contemplate your day, or the day before, depending on when you journal. If you asked yourself a Triple R day question, what was your answer? Make this as personal as you want.

7. On Sunday, look at your week in review. What did you learn? What will you do differently? What days will be your Triple R days next week?

8. Share the journal with your buddy and mentor. This can be done on a program like Google Docs or the online buddy and mentoring program offered at www.2dayGift.com/Mentoring.

Christie's journal

This is Christie's actual daily journal. The first week is day by day. Weeks 2-8 are Triple R days and weekly summaries of Christie's daily journals which are located in the Resources section. You can read as she progresses and learns to change her life patterns and wellness. She is still living the UdP principles with her husband and demonstrating the sustainability of the process. Her last diet (before UdP), was her last diet.

Congratulations, Christie!

Journal Week #1 – First week on UdP

Monday - Regular Day

Breakfast	Protein shake - almond milk/banana/protein powder/spinach/maca blend (chia/maca/cacao nibs)/peanut butter
	Green tea - 20 oz
Lunch	Salad with greens/corn/black beans/salsa/chicken
Snack	Organic dark chocolate w/sea salt and almonds - 2 squares
	½ of total bar (8 squares)
Dinner	Baked salmon w/rub - 5.5 oz
	Roasted asparagus w/olive oil, garlic salt, pepper - 6 spears
	Few bites of roasted chicken while prepping for tomorrow's soup

	Seltzer water with a splash of organic tart cherry juice and ½ lime - 12 oz
Fluids consumed	Water (includes seltzer, not tea) - 48 oz
Supplements	Vit D3 5000 IU, turmeric 450mg 2XDay, Omega 3 1280mg, Zyrtek, CoQ10 100mg, Acidophilus 2XDay, BP Meds Norvasc 7.5mg/day
Weight	212.0
Slept	1:00am - 6am 5 hours
Physical Activity	Went for a 2.72 walk 18.53 minute mile total time 51.18
Notes	Woke up feeling very excited about this journey. Meditated for 15 minutes after waking up as I have every morning since 1/1/16. Journal writing after meditation For now, keeping track of portions because I know that in the past this has been an issue, not letting my body signal when it is full. Instead eating bigger portions/2nd helpings Practiced mindful eating - not doing something else while eating. TV was on in the background but I was not on my computer.

Tuesday - Triple R day		**Calories**
Breakfast	Protein shake	
	Almond milk - 4 oz	20
	Banana - ½	50

	Protein powder - 1 T	75
	Spinach - 1 cup	20
	Maca blend - 1 T	35
	Green Tea - 20 oz	0
	Total	**200**
Lunch	Chicken soup	
	Rotisserie chicken breast no skin - 3 oz	130
	Mushrooms- ½ c	10
	Bok choy - 1 c	0
	Bean sprouts - 1 c	10
	Zucchini - 1 c	20
	Fire roasted tomatoes -½ c	30
	Chicken broth - 1 c	10
	Total	**220**
Snack	1 mini sea salt/almond chocolate wafer	15
	Total	**15**
Dinner	Sweet potato - ½ microwaved	60
	Butter - 1 t	25
	Black beans - ¼ cup	60
	Grapes - 4	10
	Mac 'n' cheese - 4 spoonfuls	100
	Total	**255**
Grand Total Day Calories		**690**
Fluids consumed	Water - 40 oz (does not include tea)	

Supplements	Vit D3 5000 IU, turmeric 450mg 2XDay, Omega 3 1280mg, Zyrtek, CoQ10 100mg, Acidophilus 2XDay, BP Meds Norvasc 7.5mg/day
Weight	210.4
Slept	11:30pm - 7am 7.5 hours
Physical Activity	None
Hours/Calorie Red	8pm - 9am 4 + 24 + 9 = 37
Notes	Woke up feeling great, excited, grounded 15 min meditation Journal writing - answered one of the 104 questions Realized I did not eat as much of the soup as I had intended. Still including the calorie count for what I intended to eat. By the time I got home, realized I was very hungry so changed the way I was going to prepare dinner. Found myself becoming irritable so popped some grapes into my mouth. Also realized that when preparing food for my son, I usually taste it, hence the mac 'n' cheese bites. Had I been not as hungry and frustrated, I think I would have been able to not have any. Although I went over the 600 (possibly) I decided to keep it a Triple R day as I was doing lots of self-analysis on why I eat and when I eat. Was feeling some doubt and feelings of self sabotage, but worked through them. No room for guilt on a Triple R day. That is not the point.

Respect the Triple R days. I love this program for so many reasons, but the big one is that, for me it addresses the mind/body/spirit connection. I am so ready for this in my life.

Wednesday - Regular Day

Breakfast	Protein shake - almond milk/banana/protein powder/spinach/maca blend(chia/maca/cacao nibs)/peanut butter
	Green tea - 20 oz
Lunch	Gluten free pizza - olive oil base/chic breast/mushrooms/artichoke hearts - 2 small pieces
Snack	Mini sea salt/almond chocolate wafers - 4
Snack	Chocolate covered strawberries - 2
	Mango - 2 slices
	Kiwi - ½
	Cantaloupe - 2 small pieces
Dinner	Sweet potato w/butter - ½
	Black beans - ½ c
	Mac 'n' cheese - ½ c
	Avocado - ½
	Seltzer water w/cherry juice and lime
Snack	Pistachios - handful
	Ravioli - 1
	Pork chop - 2 slices

Fluids consumed	Water (includes seltzer, not tea) - 36 oz
Supplements	Vit D3 5000 IU, turmeric 450mg 2XDay, Omega 3 1280mgZyrtek, CoQ10 100mg, Acidophilus 2XDay, BP Meds Norvasc 7.5mg/day
Weight	209.4
Slept	11:30pm - 7am 7.5 hours
Physical Activity	Went for a 2.71 walk 18.29 minute mile total time 50.03
Notes	Feeling much better today. Took a sleeping supplement last night,magnesium plus some other natural supplements. Don't usually sleep well. Paying attention to body signals regarding when I am starting to feel full. Also, examining my need for late night snacking. Not sure why I felt I needed to have a snack at 9:30 last night. Excited about tomorrow's Triple R to see how I do compared to Tuesday's Triple R day.

Thursday - Triple R day		**Calories**
Breakfast	Protein shake	200
	Green tea - 20 oz	
	Total	**200**

Lunch	Chicken soup	220
	Total	**220**
Snack	Mini sea salt/almond chocolate wafer - 1	15
	Grape - 1	3
	Total	**18**
Dinner	Turkey burger - 4 oz raw	90
	Broccoli - ½ c	15
	Olive oil - 1 t	40
	Parmesan - 1 T	20
	Total	**165**
Grand Total Day Calories		**603**

Fluids consumed Water - 40 oz (does not include tea)/cup choco rooibos tea

Supplements Vit D3 5000 IU, turmeric 450mg 2XDay, Omega 3 1280mg, Zyrtek, CoQ10 100mg, Acidophilus 2XDay, BP Meds Norvasc 7.5mg/day

Weight 209.4

Slept 1:00am - 7am 6.0 hours

Physical Activity None

Hours/Calorie Red 9:30pm - 9am 2.5 + 24 + 9 = 34.5

Notes Mid-afternoon I found myself feeling very hungry, which is where the snack came in handy. Still figuring out food planning and adjusting

Other than hunger, I am feeling pretty good physically. I also realize how important sleep is. I did not get enough last night and I can feel it today.

Friday – Regular Day

Breakfast	Protein shake - almond milk/protein powder/spinach/maca blend(chia/maca/cacao nibs)/peanut butter/kiwi/pineapple/strawberries
	Green tea - 20 oz
Lunch	Sweet potato w/butter - ½
	Roasted broccoli w/olive oil & parm - ½ c
	Black beans - ½ c
	Avocado - ½
	Rotisserie chicken leg/thigh - few bits
Snack	Dark chocolate - 2 squares
Dinner	Marinated hanger steak - 4.5 oz
	Garlic bread - 2 pieces
	Corn w/butter - 1 ear
	Seltzer water with cherry juice/lime
Fluids consumed	Water - 44 oz (includes seltzer, not tea)
Supplements	Vit D3 5000 IU, turmeric 450mg 2XDay, Omega 3 1280mg, Zyrtek, CoQ10 100mg, Acidophilus 2XDay, BP Meds Norvasc 7.5mg/day

Weight 207.4

Slept 12:30am - 9:30am 9 hours

Physical Activity Went for a 2.72 walk 18.16 minute mile total time 49.43

Notes Noticing I feel like I want to eat healthy. Although this process is not focused on weight loss, I am feeling inspired by the few pounds I have lost so far as well as the overall feeling of wellbeing. I am not craving junk food or feeling like the glass or two of wine that usually accompanies my weekend nights. Still lots of emotions coming up in regards to what it means to me to be healthy in mind/body/spirit

Saturday Regular Day

Breakfast Granola w/almond milk - ⅓ c

Grapes - handful

Bacon - 5 slices

Mango - ½

Scrambled eggs w/cheese/onion/bell pepper sautéed in a little butter/olive oil - small portion

Green tea - 20 oz

DandyBlend beverage w/splash creamer - 1 c

Snack Movie theater popcorn w/butter

Lunch Thai shrimp salad/slice banana cheesecake

Dinner Marinated hanger steak - 1 oz

	Ham luncheon meat - 1 piece
	Pistachios - handful
	Cole slaw - a few bites
	Choco covered strawberry - 1
	Mac 'n' cheese - 1 c
	Chocolate rooibos tea - 1 c
Fluids consumed	32 oz (not including tea)
Supplements	Vit D3 5000 IU, turmeric 450mg 2XDay, Omega 3 1280mg, Zyrtek, CoQ10 100mg, Acidophilus 2XDay, BP Meds Norvasc 7.5mg/day
Weight	207.8
Slept	12:30am - 9:30am 9 hours
Physical Activity	None
Notes	We celebrated Father's Day today instead of tomorrow so went out to the movies and lunch. Still feeling like I want to stay on the healthy eating path so I was mindful of my portions and my food choices. I chose not to drink alcohol at lunch but did not deprive myself of dessert. Drank water instead.

Journal Week #2 (located in Resources Section)

CHAPTER 9

Buddies and mentors

Why have UdP buddies and a mentor?

I consider having UdP buddies and a mentor so important that I devoted 25% of my principles to them. Achieving your ideal weight isn't like other issues. For instance if you smoke and you want to quit, all you have to do is stop. I know that's simplifying the issue, because there is actual chemical, social, and habitual addiction with smoking tobacco. But you know when you have completed that task because you have stopped smoking. It's the same with drinking alcohol.

But losing weight to reach and maintain your ideal is different, because you can't stop eating. You can change what you eat and you can use a process like the UdP, but you have to eat. Not only that, but the years of yo-yo dieting has put your desire to lose weight at odds with your body wanting to protect itself from your fad diets.

Add to this your *years* of bad eating habits. It could be you've had issues with dysfunctional eating. Perhaps the issues don't rise to the level of eating disorders, but you have destructive eating and drinking behaviors that are ingrained in your personal, social, and professional life. Maybe you occasionally binge drink, are prone to depression, are frustrated by failed prior weight loss attempts, or are just plain scared.

A buddy can help with those feelings of failure. A mentor can suggest proven strategies to cope with behaviors or at least point you in the correct direction if it's out of their area of expertise. Buddies and a mentor are there for you and are committed to your success. Remember, the diet industry is a $670 billion dollar marketing and sales organization - do you really want to tackle that alone?

UdP was uniquely designed to use buddies and a mentor

The UdP is process oriented. Because it is not content driven, you and your buddy can do the same program but eat completely different foods at different times. You can have Triple R days on different days and still support each other. You both enjoy the benefits of the Triple R day. You both understand the terminology. You both understand that weight loss is a side benefit of healthy habits. In short you can be a mirror to each other, reflecting what's best in your partner back to each other.

With UdP, you and your buddy can travel the same path together – independently.

UdP was designed to be simple. But that doesn't mean it's easy - especially at the beginning. If you start together, you can grow together as you learn the system. If you join an online mentoring program you can grow with a community of people all traveling the same path. This interaction makes you accountable and increases the likelihood of success four-fold.

There is plenty of research on the benefits of having a buddy and being accountable. In one case study, an obese woman directly attributed her success, *this time*, to her sister and her coach (Stelter, 2015). She hired a coach because she was so tired of dieting on her own. Her weight loss was good, but imagine the success if she had multiple buddies on a system that didn't focus on weight loss but on getting healthier.

Looking at the model of the body as an open system, recall that wellness (ideal weight as an indicator) occurs in quadrant 1 (Q1) with the body and mind in sync. So, when change occurs, the body and mind can begin to drift (Q2). If nothing is done, the mind and body get seriously out of sync (Q3) and require a UdP reset (Q4) to move back to wellness.

The Body's Reaction to Stress

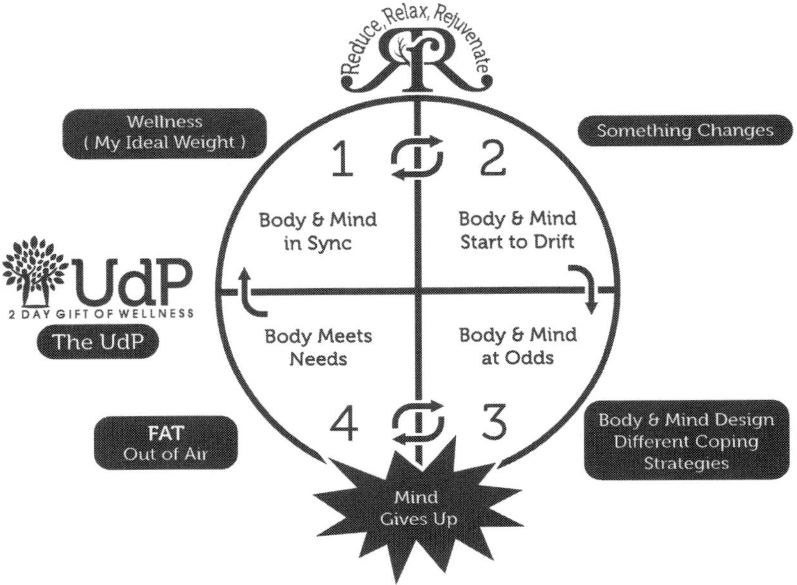

Get a free color chart that you can download here:
www.2dayGift.com/gifts

Buddies and a mentor help you make that transition, but more importantly they help you stay in Q1 by working with you when change occurs in Q2. Once you have reached your ideal weight and optimum wellness, buddies and a mentor can help you stay in the top half of the model, never letting your body and mind drift too far.

MacLean noted in a 2015 study in *Obesity Review* that dieting awakens the body's defense system, employing a well-focused, all-encompassing effort to restore the body's fat. That's what is occurring in the bottom half of the model (Q3 and Q4). The bottom half is also where yo-yo dieting happens. The UdP is designed to stop that cycle. The 8 principles are intended to solve the metabolic syndrome that Dulloo & Montani (2015) suggested leads to weight regain and obesity.

The more important a call or action is to our soul's evolution, the more resistance we feel towards pursuing it - Steven Pressfield

---

This is a macro or high-level view of why UdP uses buddies and a mentor to move to wellness, or maintain wellness, which is the ultimate goal of UdP. On a day-to-day basis, research shows that "an unconventional 'low tension' strategy [like UdP] may offer effective support of stable, long-term changes well integrated in everyday life."(Hansen, et al., 2014). More importantly, UdP is a sustainable process which MacLean suggests is required to counter these sustained and persistent attempts at weight loss.

One of the hallmarks of the UdP is that the process helps overcome personal resistance. We know we need to increase our wellness. We want to increase our wellness. We might even be ready, but it's hard to do the most important things, because of fear of failure. For instance, "What if I fail at this life-improving, life-extending process? What does that say about me?"

Here is a simple way to decide if you are resisting. Check yourself now (and again during any Triple R day) for any of these resistance disguises:

- Fear
- Self-doubt
- Procrastination
- Addiction
- Distraction

- Timidity
- Self-loathing
- Perfectionism

Pressfield (2002) believes resistance is the most toxic force. It's what keeps us from doing that which would improve our life and wellbeing. Resistance is what keeps the writer from sitting down to write. Resistance keeps the UdP client from respecting the Triple R day, even when he or she knows this well-thought -out process brings together all the elements of ideal weight and wellness. Get over resistance with buddies, accountability, and a mentor.

Kinds of UdP buddies

There are many different kinds of UdP buddies. Each of these types brings somethings unique to the table. We will concentrate on the domestic animal: friends/family members, coworkers, and online communities. The problem with buddies that are not familiar with the UdP is that they confuse this with a diet. Because they confuse it, they support you as if it's a diet by focusing on your weight loss goals. No matter how much you explain weight loss is a side effect of the 8 principles, they still measure you and your success by how much weight you lose. One buddy who does not have that issue is the domestic pet.

Kushner (2008) wrote in *Obesity Management*, the first question you should ask a patient who is overweight is, "Do you have a dog?" That's how important he felt about the social support a domestic animal provides. They give unconditional love and acceptance. They don't care if your wellness journey is taking too long, or that you had a setback. They encourage you to walk, jog or just play. My doctor, who had lost 100 pounds on a "medical diet" told me he had gained 25 pounds back in the last few months. He swears it was because his dog died. He was depressed and had no one to walk with him, so resistance raised its ugly head.

Friends, family members, and coworkers make up the next group of buddies. They know us and support us. Although I don't recommend the UdP for children without a medical doctor's agreement because of growth spurts, parents do model good wellness behaviors. Children learn by watching their parents and may change harmful attitudes about themselves as they see their parents do likewise (Berry et al, 2014). At work, employers or health care providers might support wellness programs, which are ideal venues for finding a buddy.

The most researched buddy is the romantic partner. There are good reasons for having your romantic partner be your buddy and some negative reasons. According to Jackson & Steptoe (2015), if you involve your romantic partner in behavior changes [UdP] they might help improve your outcomes. Your best chance for a positive outcome is if your partner is ready for change and joins you on his or her own UdP journey.

But the partner who "supports" you may be helpful or harmful, depending on a variety of issues. If they want to change their diets in the same direction as you are, that's good. If they are unwilling, they may support you, but sabotage you at the same time. For instance, it's helpful if they may remind you that candy is high in calories and not consistent with your stated desire to eat healthier food. But if they eat the bag of candy in front of you, that's not supportive.

If they go to the gym with you, that's helpful. If they watch your young children while you go to the gym, that's helpful. If they complain about all the time you are spending working out, yet don't want to go to the gym, that's not helpful (Theis, Carpenter, & Leustek, 2016). If your partner does the shopping and buys and prepares food that works for your Triple R day or regular day meals, that's helpful. If they buy food that sabotages your Triple R day, it's not.

For the UdP journey, romantic partners are a mixed bag. The best-selling points for having buddies, partners, coworkers, and family members for the UdP is that you can travel the same journey together, yet independently. Diets require constant restriction of calories, food types, eating times, exercise, or purchasing special foods. The UdP requires none of that. You only count calories twice a week, and eat regular, although mindful, meals the rest of the week. At most you inconvenience your family members and partners twice a week.

Online buddies

Social media provides a new way of using the buddy system. There are many online opportunities to connect with a buddy to do the UdP program. One example is Google Docs. If you post your journal online and invite other people in the UdP program to view and make comments, you can mentor and even support other people. I used this method with my first test groups. Later I added mass email, weekly video chats, and finally a dedicated Facebook page for a test group of UdP participants.

The UdP can be successfully completed by an individual. I'm an example of someone who completed the program without any help. But the research and my clients confirm that the process is much easier, and has a greater chance of success, with a support group. From my test groups I discovered that groups:

- Help create a sense of community
- Solve problems together
- Contribute by describing the process
- Encourage cheerleading!

Mass email was efficient for getting information out to everyone in the group. I never really knew, however, who read them and if they understood the message. Emails get accidently deleted and even marked as spam. I didn't know if I missed emails either. I needed more information about the groups' progress, so I instituted weekly video chats.

The weekly video chats were excellent for presenting new information and getting instant feedback on how my information was being received. It was great for doing the weekly check-ins. I had two observations. First, I discovered that each week, fewer people showed up for the weekly check-in because of prior commitments, time zone issues, discomfort with video, not wanting to "get ready" for a video conference, etc. Second, weekly check-ins often weren't enough.

So now I was using Google Docs, mass emails, and weekly check-ins. I added a dedicated Facebook page for each group. This worked well for some, but there was no accountability. I never knew who had looked at the content unless they commented on them. Also, it seemed that the same people responded to the posts. I put weekly check-up meetings on the site, but still had to send out mass emails or someone would miss. These multiple methods were cumbersome, to say the least, for both the clients and myself. They were also very limiting for peer coaching and encouragement.

From my studies, I knew that daily accountability is important to attaining goals. Our goal is wellness, and we use weight as a data point. We journal daily, so I could check up on everyone's progress each day on Google Docs, (as long as they journaled that day). Some of the participants kept notes on their phone and added to the journals on a weekly basis. Daily accountability was missing from my mentoring.

For the UdP to be maximized, I had to find a buddy and mentor system that was online, efficient, allowed for peer coaching and encouragement, was not time zone specific, had daily accountability built in, and was easy for the mentor and the UdP buddies. I found one, and although a complete explanation is outside the scope of this book, I would encourage you to check out www.2dayGift.com/Mentoring and sign up for the online coaching program. I believe this program will make the UdP almost fool-proof. It provides the mentoring and community involvement that will help each client get past the resistance that is sure to crop up in the first few weeks. The UdP is simple, but not easy at first.

Buddies and mentors are critical to successfully completing the UdP. Having a buddy, family member, co-worker, or romantic partner do the program with you (although independently) will greatly increase your chance for success. To optimize your chances, join the online coaching group. You don't have to take this wellness journey alone – enlist a buddy!

CHAPTER 10

Exercise

There is no principle so misapplied as exercise. It's common sense to think that calories in equal calories out. The research, however, doesn't support this simple notion. There is no causal connection between calories consumed and calories expended. Because there is no causal relationship, you must make this important paradigm shift. You have to resist the marketing blitzes that tie exercise to weight loss.

Saying that [people] lose weight because they expend more calories than they consume is like saying that students are late for class because they arrive after the bell rings. Both statements are true, but neither is causal. – Lucan & DiNicolantonio (2015).

Resisting the conventional wisdom is important for a couple of reasons. But most importantly, exercise is important on its own. You can lose weight without exercising and you can get in better shape without losing weight. So, this chapter is about severing the tie that binds exercise and weight loss.

I recently ran into an old friend. He asked me if I had been keeping in touch with a mutual friend, Robert (not his real name). I told him, "No, we were Facebook friends, but recently when I searched for him, I couldn't find him." He proceeded to tell me that Robert had passed recently.

I was shocked because Robert had been a fitness nut. He religiously left work at 4:15, after exactly 8 hours on the clock. From work he always went to the gym – always. It didn't matter if the General wanted a briefing today, at 5pm. He'd work until 4:15 and hand the incomplete briefing to one of the other members of the staff who were military and couldn't leave. I was amazed at his ability to compartmentalize and his results were impressive.

Robert's total body fat was in the single digits. He wasn't big and he never used performance enhancing drugs. He was just super fit. Robert was also 5 years younger than me, and I felt fat by comparison, even though I was in my 30s and a military officer. Robert was that fit.

So I was surprised to hear of his passing. I can remember his contagious laugh and happy outlook on life, a life that he molded around exercise. But even being fit did not protect him from the cancer that took his life so prematurely. His fitness might have helped him cope better. I don't know for sure because I didn't realize he was sick.

Do I tell this story to demonstrate how exercise is worthless? No, on the contrary. The research shows that if you are obese and out of shape and you can only do one activity, lose weight or exercise, the choice is clear – exercise. As I will explain later, the benefits of exercise are many, but weight loss is a side benefit, not the main reason to exercise. Like every principle, the exercise principle needs to be viewed from the perspective of wellness and sustainability.

Robert's total commitment to exercise is not sustainable for the majority of the population. Exercise is an important piece of the holistic wellness system, but it cannot stand alone. For exercise to be sustainable, it has to be enjoyable for the person exercising. Before we can discuss what exercises are best, I'd like to define exercise as I use it.

Calories in (eating) minus calories out (exercise) has never worked, long term, in the history of weight loss.

There are two types of exercise – intentional exercise and inadvertent exercise. Intentional exercise is structured, usually in duration and type. Inadvertent exercise is generally termed "physical activity" by researchers. Inadvertent exercise might be walking your dog. The activity you enjoy is being with your dog and your dog enjoys going for a walk. So, in order to be with your dog you go on a walk. Intentional exercise takes place in the gym, often with a set routine, such as abs on Monday and Friday; lower body on Tuesday, etc. The purpose of intentional exercise is to get in shape or maintain fitness.

The difference is important because we only do inadvertent exercise on the Triple R days. After the first few weeks of the program, I recommend beginning an intentional exercise program with sustainability as the goal. If you are currently involved with an intentional exercise program, I recommend you continue on regular days (non-Triple R day). In essence, your Triple R days are days of rest from intentional exercise. Remember, the Triple R days are for Reducing (stress and calories), Relaxing, and allowing your body to Rejuvenate.

If you are an exercise enthusiast, like I am, I ask you to put away your bias about exercise and weight loss for a little while. I ask you to try to complete the paradigm shift in *exercise – diet - lose weight mentality*. Shift to "exercise has weight loss as a *possible side effect*" (if used correctly). The paradigm shift also requires that you lose, at least for the moment, the "no pain - no gain; more is better mentality" of excessive exercising, at least as used in weight loss or maintenance.

Most people believe that exercise leading to weight loss is always good. Researchers know differently. There is a phenomenon known as "the obesity paradox." The obesity paradox really points out obesity bias, a completely different term. The feeling that thinner is better than fatter is *obesity bias*. The paradox of obesity is that obese individuals who are suffering from cardiovascular disease (heart disease, or CV) live longer than thin people with cardiovascular disease (Swift, et al, 2014). Thus the paradox: if thin is better (bias), then how is it that obese people with CV live longer (the paradox)? Neither the research nor I suggest that a person suffering from CV should gain weight and become obese. That's why it is a paradox. What to do?

I would say there is also an exercise bias when it comes to weight loss. Most people exercise to maintain their current weight or to lose weight. Some lucky few (in our society) exercise to gain weight. So the bias is that exercise and weight loss is tethered, even with the knowledge that most people do not sustain their weight loss even with exercise, and some people gain weight when they exercise. This tethering is best expressed in the "calories in - calories out" method of dieting and exercising.

A review of the current data in the role of exercise in weight loss in 2014 (Swift, et al) showed that exercise-driven weight loss is not likely, except with hours and hours of aerobic exercise. Coaches and personal trainers that preach this are setting their clients up for unrealistic expectations. The researchers even found that large amounts of resistance training (weight lifting) by itself is not likely to produce weight loss. There is no combination of calorie reduction and exercise that produces "likely" weight loss. This is a stunning revelation.

An in-depth review of the research in 2014 found that "unless the overall volume of aerobic [exercise] is very high, clinically significant weight loss is unlikely to occur." – Damon Swift

---

Research reveals over and over again that exercise may lead to temporary weight loss. But the body, being an open system, has creative ways to save energy when put under stress – especially the stress of exercise when tied with calorie reduction (diet). A July 2015 article in American College of Sports Medicine, titled *Physical Activity and the Missing Calories* looked at this issue. Geneticist Gene Neel theorized that we have a set of "thrifty genes" whose purpose is to get the body to store fat. Neel concluded that this gene was a result of natural selection of our hunter-gather ancestors. Of course, since we "hunt" for food with our dollars now, this gene has probably outlived its usefulness except to explain why weight loss is unsustainable, even with increased exercise.

Nothing in biology makes sense except in the light of evolution. – Theodosius Dobzhansky (famous geneticist)

Conventional wisdom (calories in, calories out) suggest the more we exercise, the more weight we will lose. Any of us who have been on diets knows intuitively that this doesn't work. We notice some people eat all the time and don't gain weight. They have a high metabolism. Other people look at ice cream and gain 5 pounds. They have slow metabolisms. Studies prove this (Pontzer, 2015). Research shows that our bodies have a set point that the body tries to maintain within a certain range. This set range is fairly narrow. We can exercise and reduce calories, but the body will change to get back to its desired weight. I call this making *fat out of air*. There are several reasons for this: biological, genetic, emotional, and stress.

That's why we look for an ideal weight when we look at a holistic approach to wellness. Your weight on the scale is just a number that provides an indication of your general health. If you notice a weight gain, you use your Triple R day to rejuvenate, but also to discover what has changed to cause your body to store fat (your rainy day fund). By discovering and resolving the issue, you allow your body to reduce the rainy day fund.

High intensity interval training [sprinting] and moderate to vigorous intensity continuous training [jogging, biking, and rowing] are both effective in improving heart health. High intensity, however is more enjoyable, takes less time, and therefore is more sustainable.

If weight loss is just a side effect of exercise, why exercise? The bottom line is we exercise to increase our wellness. Exercise is good for your brain. Just the movement of exercise stimulates the brain to grow and replace damaged brain cells. Exercise produces endorphins which make you feel better about yourself and your body.

The physical act of exercising strengthens your bones and improves your heart health, and the fresh air can elevate your attitude. In short, we exercise because it is good for the body, mind, and soul. And a possible side effect is weight loss. That's not just because of the increased calorie burn, but because the increased wellness allows your body to use fat and not replace it. There's no longer a need for your body to store the same amount of fat.

The research shows you can have different results from exercise based on the type, duration, and intensity. Conventional wisdom says extended periods of moderate aerobic exercise, such as jogging, swimming and biking will burn the most fat. The studies show different results. When I looked at exercise, the most important factor was health and sustainability. Few people can jog or even walk three times a week for five miles. On January 1st of every year, millions of people make resolutions to do that, but by February very few are still exercising, after being sidelined by injury or lack of motivation.

Research by Clark, (2015), Bouchonville et al (2014), and Kong et al (2016) suggests that short duration, high intensity workouts have the same effect as longer, more moderate exercise. The good news is that high intensity isn't the same for everyone. If you are Michael Phelps, your interval training level is different from mine. But as my health improves, so does the intensity of my training.

This is where your doctor and personal trainer come in. After a thorough check-up from your doctor, hire a personal trainer to help you develop a high intensity interval training program for both aerobic (sprinting) and resistance training (weight lifting).

An example of an aerobic workout would be to walk five minutes, warming up at a slow pace. You can literally do this anywhere, even during your lunch break at work. You will sweat some doing this workout so you may have to change your shirt if you're at work. But you're not going to sweat like you were running five miles because you're not getting that heated. After you walk for 5 minutes, do a quick jog for 30 seconds. A quick jog will be different for each person, but for me it is about a 10-minute pace – it's not very fast at all. Do whatever you can do that's easy. If you can only do a 12-minute pace or a 15-minute pace, then do that slow jog or trot. You're still doing a warm up. You do it for 30 seconds, and then rest by fast walking for 1 minute.

Then you do it again. But this time start the jog faster (9 minute mile) for 30 seconds. You're still warming up your heart, legs, and tendons for running. Then fast walk for a minute. That's a minute and a half total. Next you do another 30-second jog, a little faster than the last one, and fast walk for a minute.

Of course, you will catch your breath and your heart rate will decrease, but your heart rate doesn't go down to a resting rate because there's not enough time.

Now you start your sprints. The sprints are basically five sprints for 30 seconds, with a minute and a half walking in between. You've increased the time off to a minute and a half. During the five sprints, you are running as fast as you can until your 30 seconds is up. When the 30 second sprint is completed, just slowly decrease your speed to a walk again for a minute and a half. Repeat four more times. At the end of the 5th sprint, walk another 5 minutes to cool down. But whenever you need to cool down, you can just go back to work. This takes about 20 minutes in total. You can do this three times a week. That's less than an hour a week, and you get all the aerobic exercise you would do if you ran three or four miles a couple of times a week, without the damage to your knees and other joints.

Aerobic interval training (19 minutes)

5 minute walk
30 second slow jog
1 minute walk
30 second faster jog
1 minute walk
30 second faster jog
1 minute walk

30 second sprint
1.5 minute walk
Repeat the sprint and walk 4 more times (5 total)
5 minute cool down walk

That's an example of an aerobic exercise. You do the same concept with resistance training (weight lifting). Again, use a professional trainer if you don't have the experience to do this alone. The concept is the same as with running. Your goal is to exercise your muscles to the point of fatigue with little rest in between. You pick 10 exercises that target different parts of your body and for 30 seconds you lift as much weight as you can. If you finish your 30 seconds and aren't tired, next time pick up the pace or increase the weight. But for now, move on to the next exercise. Do one 30-second set per exercise. After the 30 seconds, rest for 1 minute.

Resistance training (weight lifting) – 9 minutes

5 minute walk
2 minute warmup of jump rope or jumping jacks
30 seconds of shoulder presses
1 minute rest
30 seconds of bicep curls
1 minute rest
Repeat this pattern for the remaining exercises
Romanian dead lift
Push up
Sit up (crunch)
Alternating lunges
Squats
Dips
Bent over row

Burpee
2 minute walk around to cool down

Form is important for resistance training. Don't lift too fast or too much weight. You don't want to injure yourself. Different exercise requires different weight, based on your ability. I highly recommend a personal trainer or an experienced partner when you do resistance training. Forget *no pain – no gain*. That's not what we are after here, unless you are a serious athlete and are training for an event like a marathon. You know your own body, so don't injure yourself. Above is an example of what a 9-minute workout would look like. Do this a couple of times a week and soon your muscle definition and strength will improve.

To summarize, you exercise to increase your wellness. Weight loss is a welcome side-effect if you are above your ideal body weight. Resist the temptation to work out harder or longer just to lose weight. That approach does not work - it's not sustainable. Sever the tether between exercise and weight loss. Only do exercises you like and switch them up. The two examples are effective training routines, but get a trainer to help you. Remember, don't do these exercises on Triple R days. Only do stretching style yoga or inadvertent exercise (walking the dog, taking a leisurely hike, etc). Learn to enjoy your new wellness. Do not injure yourself.

CHAPTER 11

UdP on the road

The travelers' guide

As an international airline captain, I cross the globe constantly. You might think this would wreak havoc with the UdP program, but it actually didn't require any adjustments to the process. This section will look at how I was able to lose the 25 pounds while traversing multiple countries and continents. I will also include the comments and observation of Larry, an international pilot flying the MD-11. His weight loss was similar to mine, as you'll read about soon. Keep in mind that weight loss is a by-product of healthy living, so how do you do that when you travel?

I have found the UdP process to be extremely valuable to my health. The Triple R days are more challenging because I am not allowed to take food off the airplane or carry a cooler to bring my own food. So I have to shop the local economy. This is where the UdP is far superior to any conventional diet.

With a conventional diet you have to keep track of calories or points, or eat certain types of food. With the UdP, I only count calories 2 days a week. Those two days can be challenging, but the rest of the time I can eat anything I enjoy, as long as I do it mindfully. That simplifies the food issues significantly. Who wants to eat packed food when you travel internationally? Not Larry or me, we want to experience life. Once you incorporate the UdP into your life, you'll be amazed that when you travel internationally, you do not gain weight. You might actually lose some. You will also be less susceptible to foreign viruses or bacteria.

Larry's and my experiences were mostly international travel, but we did have some domestic trips and both of us agree that domestic is much easier. For the business traveler, the UdP is probably the only way to stay healthy on road trips. For the vacation traveler, both clients and I have reported losing weight or gaining very little weight on vacation. When is the last time that happened to you?

Here is a musing from my book *Ballet in a Coal Mine* (2017):

A Week in Advance

On a deadhead flight from Singapore,
A casual conversation turned serious;
Asking questions never dared before.

If I told you that you were to die next week,
What would you change?
Nothing, I only plan a week in advance.

Business travelers and pilots have plans that change at a moment's notice. Pilots, for instance, often don't know their schedules more than a week or two in advance, which makes planning almost impossible. I have to confess that the UdP lifestyle takes planning, specifically the Triple R day. But the health benefits and the ability to fight off jet lag more than make up for the planning. Let me begin with Larry's story.

Larry's story

I am a retired USAF fighter pilot and a current airline pilot flying mostly long-haul, international routes. I'm 57 years old. I've kept myself in decent shape physically over the years by hitting the hotel gyms almost daily when on layovers. However, over the last three years, my weight has slowly crept up pound by pound, and the large shifts in time zones have taken their toll on my desire to work out regularly. My energy levels were such that I spent most of my layovers lounging around instead of working out or even going for long walks in the international cities where we stay. Feeling old? You bet.

Then I flew a two-week Asia trip with Dr. (Captain) Mike Christensen as he was in the final stages of developing the Ultimate diet Process. We discussed in detail his extensive research and findings as well as the concepts behind the UdP. Those concepts are so simple and easy to follow: eat when you are hungry (don't eat when you are not hungry), drink when you are thirsty, sleep when you are sleepy, and respect the Triple R days. If you exercise, do it for better health, not to lose weight. Weight is a data point, not a goal. Better health is the goal.

Near the end of that trip, Mike asked me if I wanted to be a tester for the UdP. As I mentioned above, my overall health had been in decline over several years and I needed to do something to reverse that decline. I had just sat through a two-week crash course with the author of UdP and fully agreed with everything he said, so of course I wanted to be one of his testers. The test involved following the program, keeping a daily journal and reporting weekly on what I ate, how I felt, providing occasional weight measurements, and attending weekly a videoconference with Mike and the other people in the test, when my schedule allowed.

I just completed the 12-week UdP beta test with my last week spent in the mountains of Idaho hunting elk. In the 12 weeks, I lost 25 pounds in total with 10 pounds going away quickly and then a slow but fairly steady reduction over the rest of the test. I came to enjoy RRR days, and sometimes ate at the end of the RRR day just to get my calorie count up to 600 even though I wasn't really hungry.

The only difficult thing for me as an international airline pilot was trying to fit the concept of a RRR "day" into my schedule when crossing up to 12 time zones at a time, as well as going back and forth over the International Date Line. Mike, being intimately familiar with that problem, came up with an easy solution of basing the "day" on the 24-hour period before the next flight instead of the normal calendar day I used at home.

What do I think about the UdP? This is the best thing I have done for my overall health in a long, long, time. I mentioned the 25 pound weight loss but that's not important as weight is a data point, not a goal. The proof in the pudding for me is the increased energy I had this week on my elk hunting trip. A typical day for us begins with a 4:30 am wake up, a 3-5 mile morning hike between 7500 and 9500 feet elevation with 25 pounds of gear, followed by a similar hike in the afternoon. Then we get 6-7 hours of sleep and another 4:30 wake up, repeated several times.

I found climbing the hills much easier than in years past, even to the point of putting my much younger (and lighter) hunting partner, who works out extensively in preparation for hunting season, to shame. I was less winded going up the hills, had good balance going back down, never felt exhausted, and my joints never hurt as they did in years past.

Another side benefit I noticed was lack of heartburn. Before I started the beta test, I had frequent heartburn/reflux that was uncomfortable during the day and sometimes interrupted my sleep at night. I have had no episodes in the 12 weeks since I started the program.

> I'm 57 years old now, and after following the UdP for the past 12 weeks, I feel better than I have in years. The concepts are simple and easy to follow and I believe the process will be easy to sustain for the rest of my life. If you are looking to improve your health and quality of life, I highly recommend jumping on the UdP bandwagon. I want to thank Dr. Mike Christensen for his extensive research into diet programs that fail time after time, and for developing a better alternative for healthier living, the Ultimate diet Process.

Larry's story validates how it is possible to get healthy while traveling for 2 weeks a month. Larry's weight loss was 25 pounds, but what he gained was energy, stamina, better sleep, and less acid reflux. Personally, I noticed my plantar fasciitis slowly went away as well as a shoulder injury repairing without physical therapy. The problems and injuries slowly disappeared over time. For instance I observed after a few months that I didn't suffer from sinus headaches because of the airplane air or the Texas summer. One day I just realized I hadn't taken any allergy pills in weeks and couldn't remember the last sinus headache. At my last flight physical my weight had dropped 25 pounds from six month previous to that, plus my blood pressure had lowered to 107/79. Not bad for a 60 year old man.

Let's get started on how the principles work when *we are on the road again*. If you recall, the eight principles of wellness that are designed into the Ultimate diet Process (UdP) are:

1. Sustainability
2. Eat when you're hungry
3. Eat mindfully
4. Respect the Triple R day
5. Journal every day
6. The buddy system

7. Find a mentor
8. Exercise

Remember, the principles are listed as single principles that combine to make the UdP. If you decide to skip one principle, you might be successful for a while, but undoubtedly you will fail in the long run.

The 8 Principles of UdP Wellness

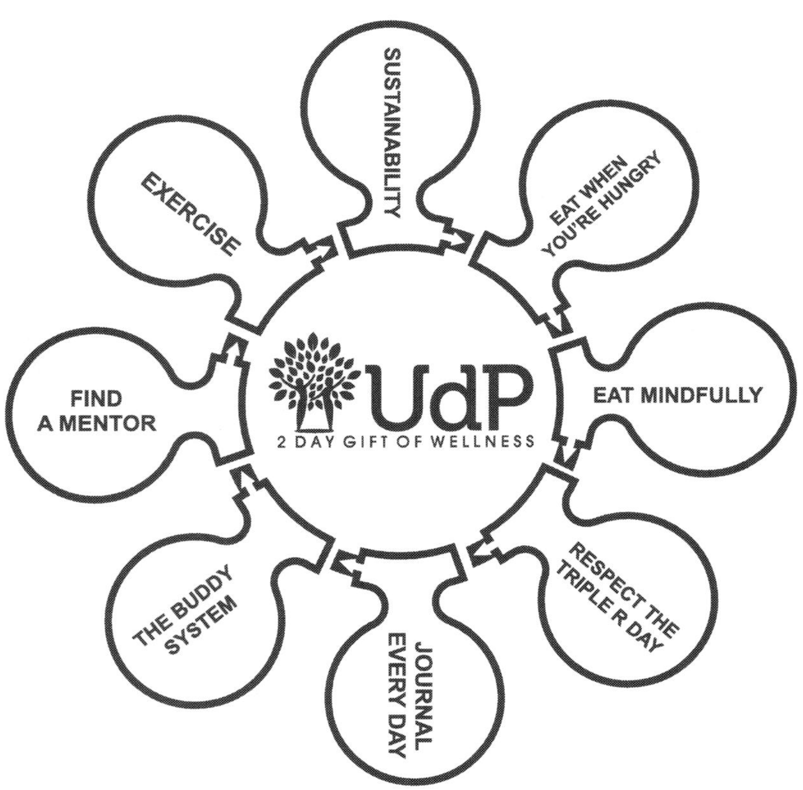

Get a free color chart that you can download here: www.2dayGift.com/gifts

Sustainability

Sustainability means staying power. The one thing all diets have in common is that they are unsustainable. If they are unsustainable they will fail. The diet industry knows that and counts on you forgetting it.

When flying internationally, you develop a rhythm. But you are not always on the road, so you need a process you can use on the road and at home. The UdP gives you flexibility to choose which days are Triple R days and which are regular days.

Eat when you're hungry

It is still very important to eat when you are hungry. Pilots and other business travelers eat when food is available. Another trap is to get the order mixed up. We are supposed to eat when we are hungry, sleep when we are tired, and drink when we are thirsty. Often, being trapped in an airplane or in some foreign town, we sleep when we are hungry, eat when we are tired, and hardly drink at all. It's no wonder our bodies are under stress while traveling!

I stepped on the scales (after my international trip) and realized I had lost almost 20 pounds in 6 weeks. I think that is a good pace that I can sustain long-term. – Larry

---

This means we need to be extra vigilant about what our body needs. We have to schedule our drinking because we know that the dry airplane air will dehydrate us. Plan to drink a few cups of water every hour. When you get up to stretch your legs to prevent deep vein thrombosis, get a bottle of water and drink all of it before your next break.

Here are some final cautions when eating on the road. Be careful not to eat out of boredom. Don't eat to fall asleep. And don't eat out of stress and loneliness. That never works.

Eat mindfully

Eating mindfully means thinking about what your brain decides to put into the body. The best thing about the UdP is that 5 days a week all you have to do is watch what you eat. There is no requirement for portion or types of food, as long as you only eat when you are hungry. The nutrition tips in Chapter 6 still apply. Make sure you are enjoying what you eat.

Continue to keep a food journal, so you can monitor your individual reactions to foods. This is especially true in foreign countries where the local customs are different than in the USA. As well, the food preparation standards might be lower, so it's important to observe how we feel as we sample new foods.

I remember having a foreign dish that was delicious, but in the middle of the night I became violently sick. Lucky for me and the crew I recovered quickly. But the dish was so tasty that the next time I went there I rationalized that something else had made me sick, and ordered the same dish. When I became violently ill once more, I figured maybe I won't eat at that restaurant in the future. Genius, I know.

Respect the Triple R day

The Triple R day is a day you choose, twice a week, to reduce, relax, and rejuvenate: the Triple R. All principles are important, but, like sustainability, this principle becomes a focus of the UdP for a number of reasons.

First, the reduction speaks to reducing calories to 600 a day, two days a week. You do not reduce calories to lose weight, but to allow your body to repair and rejuvenate. Your body can only repair when you are resting. Resting includes your digestive system. Digesting food uses a lot of energy and is a major focus of the body when you eat.

Respect the Triple R day, especially the relaxing part since you are reducing on those days. – Larry

---

Relaxing is important because if you don't relax, the reduction in calories causes stress, makes you hungry and causes the body to go into hyper mode. One rule for the "relax" of the Triple R day is to not intentionally exercise. This is one time that traveling is a blessing. We don't intentionally exercise, but you can sightsee galore, time permitting. Just don't multi-task or try to put too much into the day. You should just be strolling along the promenade in Paris, not power walking the Champs-Élysées.

The buddy system

Another sustainable feature is the buddy system. Developing healthy habits is easier and has more potential for success when you do it with someone else. (Romo & Dailey, 2014). The entire crew could be on the UdP together. You can each have different goals, food habits, work schedules, and ideas about eating organic. Remember, the UdP is not content-driven. I don't even talk about what you should eat. You eat what you enjoy.

My clients who partner up really encourage each other. They know the lingo. When they say "I'm on a Triple R Day," they instantly know what that means. Or if one says they are frustrated that their weight is fluctuating, their buddy can remind them that weight is just a data point and health is the goal.

Traveling with different schedules can be a challenge. However, using one of the online coaching platforms on www.2dayGift.com or even Google docs makes keeping up with a distant partner a piece of cake. If you travel in a group, you can get a little creative, because a buddy makes everything better. You could even recruit a fellow traveler and become their buddy and mentor.

Mentor

A mentor is different from a coach or a buddy. A coach is helpful, but if they have not *successfully* completed the process, they are mostly cheerleaders. A mentor is a cheerleader, confidant, knowledge provider, and contact when issues arise.

The most surprising aspect of the UdP is the role exercise plays in weight loss – basically zero effect. Exercise is important for overall health, but doesn't impact weight loss nearly as much as we have been led to believe all our lives. – Larry

---

All the UdP mentors at www.2dayGift.com/Mentoring have completed the program and excelled at understanding and putting the principles to work in their lives. They are committed to the UdP lifestyle and to helping as many people as they can.

Exercise

The final principle is the one most people associate with weight loss - exercise. One of the tenets of the UdP is to do healthy activities that have weight loss as a by-product. Exercise is the best example. The benefits of exercise in losing weight are mixed. For instance, research suggests if you have to choose weight loss or exercise, choose exercise. Even when obesity is a factor for future health issues, the first priority is exercise. Now wouldn't it be great if there was a process that had exercise as a principle and weight loss as a by-product?

Hopefully you can begin to understand how perfect the UdP is for travelers who want to improve their health and wellbeing. Change your life and you'll change your weight. It can be effortless if you concentrate on the correct activities and realize the scale is only a devise to give you an interesting data point on your health and wellness journey. The next section will concentrate on how I would plan the UdP for international travelers - the nuts and bolts.

The nuts and bolts of following the UdP while traveling

The UdP is simple and easy, but it takes planning. Remember, the first few weeks take some getting used to. Each person reacts to reducing calories and relaxing differently. So here is how I'd recommend implementing the UdP.

On Sunday

Pick your two Triple R days. Look at your travel or flight schedule for longer layovers and days that will be less stressful. You need to have at least 24 hours where you can eat just 600 calories. If your trip is short, the Triple R days can be before and after the trip.

That way you can just eat mindfully on your trip and the travel is not an issue.

Plan your journaling. Decide on the menu for your Triple R day. There are lots of websites with menus that come in under 600 calories. If you are traveling, hard boiled eggs have between 60 -70 calories and last for a while if you can keep them refrigerated. What you don't want is to show up on your Triple R day without a plan for eating. That's a recipe for disaster.

Keep your journal up to date. Every night, record the day's activities. We supplied a journal example in the resource section, but at the very least, record your lowest weight for the day, what food you ate, any exercise you did, and how much you slept.

The day before Triple R day

Decide on the activities you want to do on your Triple R day. Remember, reducing is only ½ the job on a Triple R day. The most import activity is to relax. This is the hardest part for most people, especially women. They seem to feel guilty just relaxing. But relaxing is important for healing the body. Without the relaxing, you can't repair and rejuvenate.

Pick activities that make you happy. Smile, tomorrow is for you! Push anything stressful from tomorrow to later.

The day of the Triple R

Meditate in the morning. Learn to meditate and start the day off right. Use a mantra and quiet your thinking. Dedicate the day to letting petty things go. Commit to a stress-free day. Commit to being happy. Commit to doing only the activities YOU want to do.

Don't multi-task. Multi-tasking is very stressful on your brain. You are really starting and stopping tasks over and over again. Don't do it.

Ditch the social media. Don't get drawn into the drama. Life can go on without you for the day. The same goes for the news. Read a book, go for a walk, get a massage or a manicure, meet friends for coffee, or play golf. Do what you enjoy without being tied to your phone or a schedule.

Manage your eating. Eat when you get hungry and don't let yourself get famished. Plan to take 100-calorie snacks when you go out so that you can eat if your energy gets low. Have fun on this day and don't stress. Eat what you enjoy, but keep track of the calories. Try to stick to your plan of 600 calories.

Manage your day as it unfolds

- Get a massage/manicure/play golf
- Skip the gym
- Enjoy the creativity
- Enjoy the extra energy
- Learn about yourself
- Have a guilt-free day
- Ask yourself one of the Triple R day questions
- Recommit to not let anything bother you

What about the other 5 days of the week?

Eat what you enjoy. Keep track of what you eat (not calories, just the type of food) for your journal. Make sure you eat mindfully and healthily if you can.

Journal every day. Keep track of your food, weight, exercise and sleep. Notice how the food you eat affects you. Note how much you like not being on a diet.

Exercise. You can exercise on these days, but realize you are doing the exercise to be healthy, not to lose weight. That way you can stop before you get hurt or exhaust yourself.

Relax. Try to relax like it was a Triple R day. Meditate during the morning or anytime in the day. Ask yourself any of the Triple R day questions.

Conclusion

That's it. I told you it was simple. The UdP is an easy concept that you can take on the road. Triple R days, which take more planning, can be done before or after a trip, if appropriate. Dieting is dangerous, but the UdP is the antidote to dieting. It's safer, more flexible, and healthier than any diet. You will notice a new you emerge within 4 weeks. The UdP is sustainable, especially for the traveler's lifestyle. You will no longer gain weight or be unhealthy just because your life is more chaotic than that of other people. The UdP works – just ask Larry!

All is well with the UdP. – Larry

CHAPTER 12

Frequently asked questions

Do I have to exercise on this program?

Exercise is very important for your health. If you had to choose between exercise and losing weight, exercising is better for you. But on Triple R days, don't do any strenuous exercise.

During the first couple of weeks of UdP, don't begin a new routine. If you already work out, exercise on your non-Triple R days. The sections on nutrition and exercise give you more ideas on both topics.

Will I lose weight on this process?

If you're at your ideal weight you won't lose. You'll maintain your weight and become healthier. If you're heavy or slightly overweight and you reduce your stress by respecting the Triple R days, you can expect to lose weight.

It depends on your body. The more you can convince it that you're not starving, and that this is the time to repair, the more weight you'll lose. Weight loss can range from not losing any weight in a week, to losing 10 pounds in one week. I lost about half a pound a day for the first month, which is a lot of weight, but I had a lot to lose.

Then it starts slowing down, but as you're losing weight you'll notice that you hit set points. Your body likes set points. You'll lose five pounds, and then bounce up two or three pounds and think nothing's happening. Then you lose two pounds for a few days in a row, and you'll be five pounds lighter again, going up and down. But over time you will lose weight.

Is the Triple R day stressful?

The goal of the program is to not be stressed. If it's stressful, you're not doing it right. The idea of the Triple R day is to reduce stress and have this relaxation carry over to the rest of the week.

Your activities to reduce and manage stress on your Triple R day may inspire you to continue on the other days. If you enjoyed reading a book or the Bible, or meditating first thing in the morning, you can continue those activities all week.

You may want to have your cup of coffee or tea and not do anything else, such as checking email. You just want to relax. It's not supposed to be stressful.

Will I be hungry?

You may feel hungry the first few weeks while you're learning the process and figure out what foods to eat during your Triple R days. Obviously, the only days you could be hungry are your Triple R days because the rest of the time you eat whatever you enjoy, mindfully.

Within the first couple of weeks, you develop a system of the foods you like. We talked about sustainability and the habits of healthy individuals, so we have to think long-term. This means finding foods you enjoy that you can eat on your Triple R days for the rest of your life. If you love vegetables, you'll have a big choice of foods to eat on Triple R days because vegetables are low in calories. If you don't, you'll have to find other foods for the 600 calories.

By the second month you shouldn't be hungry on your Triple R days. You should have figured it out. If not, you probably need to relax more so your body can repair itself. Better yet, join one of the UdP online mentor and buddies groups.

Do I need to buy any special food, or use recipes?

The answer is no. There are no special foods to eat. You eat whatever you enjoy and what feels good for your body. That's where the journaling comes in. You probably have a pretty good idea of what your body likes and doesn't like by now, but we're going to fine tune it. So you can eat anything you want, but not as much as you want.

Do I need to see a doctor before I start?

That's up to you. If you're young and healthy, you probably don't need to.

I encourage you to see your doctor if you're on medication, or if you have diabetes or any kind of medical condition such as thyroid problems. You should let your doctor monitor your process because your body will change.

People on this plan who have diabetes often decrease their insulin within the second month because their body is repairing and doesn't require as much insulin. Their weight decreases as well, and they're able to control their blood sugar better.

What do I need to know about nutrition?

Because it's process-driven instead of content-driven, you can eat whatever you enjoy. That doesn't mean you *should* eat anything you want. You should choose what's good for your body.

If your body doesn't like something, it will tell you by reacting to it, either by bloating, getting tired, or other physical discomforts. If you put something in your body that will take a lot of energy to digest, the first thing it does is start converting all the energy from your brain and muscles, and you start feeling overwhelmed and tired.

That's where journaling comes in. Journaling will help you keep track of how you react to what you eat. If you feel tired after eating certain foods, you can try something different. But you have to give your body the basic nutrients for repair.

Epilogue

What now?

One of my clients asked me, "What now?" Cheri was an unusual client because she only weighed 126.5 pounds at the beginning of the UdP. She joined because she was trying to lose that "stubborn 5 pounds". At the start I told her this wasn't a diet, but a life change and that she would have to follow the 8 principles of UdP exactly. She turned out to be one of the UdP stars. (A UdP star is someone who religiously follows the program without modification.)

A short 10 weeks later, she had lost 7 1/2 pounds. But the part she liked best was how she felt. Since she was over 50, she was excited to get her waist back. She felt her hormones were better in check. She never felt bloated. She handled stress easily. However, she felt she had reached her ideal weight and didn't want to get too skinny.

While being "too skinny" might be a condition we would all like to have, it is a concern once you reach your ideal weight. Because this is a life change, she didn't want to just stop the UdP (good decision) and lose all the positive benefits. Our discussion took several directions.

1. The nature of the UdP shouldn't allow you to get too thin, so stick with the process.

2. Don't give up the Triple R days because that is when the rejuvenating for longevity takes place. Remember, fasting is the single action we can take to increase our age AND our quality of life.

3. Hire a personal trainer to get into better shape. Muscle does weigh more than fat, and getting in shape (without hurting yourself) is an important principle (8).

If your doctor tells you, or you just feel like you are getting too skinny, the simple solution is to eat additional healthy calories on your regular, non-Triple R days. Again, respect the Triple R day.

Interestingly, commercial "diet" programs or schemes don't have this problem. No, maintaining the lost weight is their big issue. With the UdP, once you hit your ideal weight and you don't want to keep losing, have a bowl of frozen yogurt, a scoop of your favorite organic ice cream, or an extra fruit smoothie - and throw in a few teaspoons of peanut butter. Hey, you changed your life. You deserve it!

Cheri's results led to a little more drama than my simple solutions. She got engaged. There's nothing like planning a wedding to increase your stress level.

Cheri, congratulations on achieving wellness. Enjoy your wedding. The whole UdP team wishes you many happy years with your husband.

Now go and live your new life deliberately.

PART 3

Resources

Triple R day sample menus

		Calories
Breakfast	Protein shake:	
	Almond milk - 4 oz	20
	Banana - ½	50
	Protein powder - 1 T	75
	Spinach - 1 cup	20
	Macablend - 1T	35
	Green tea - 20 oz	0
	Total	**200**
Lunch	Chicken soup:	
	Rotisserie chicken breast no skin - 3 oz	130
	Mushrooms - ½ cup	10
	Bok choy - 1 cup	10
	Bean sprouts - 1 cup	10
	Zucchini - 1 cup	20
	Fire roasted tomatoes - ½ cup	30
	Chicken broth - 1 cup	10
	Total	**220**
Snack	1 mini sea salt/almond chocolate wafer	15
	Total	**15**
Dinner	Sweet potato - ½ microwaved	60
	Butter - 1 t	25
	Black beans - ¼ cup	60
	Grapes - 4	10
	Total	**255**
Grand Total Day Calories		**590**

		Calories
Breakfast	Granola - ⅓ c	120
	Almond milk - ½ c	20
	Cherries - 6	60
	Green tea - 20 oz	0
	Total	**200**
Lunch	Mexican casserole - ½ c - recipe	180
	Total	**180**
Dinner	Asparagus - 5 spears	15
	Baked tofu 3 oz/olive oil - 1 t	120
	Marinated flank steak - 1 oz	60
	Peach iced tea - herbal	0
	Total	**195**
Grand Total Day Calories		**575**

		Calories
Breakfast	Protein shake	200
	Green tea - 20 oz	0
	Total	**200**
Lunch	Cauliflower - ½ c	
	Brussel sprouts - ½ cup	20
	Olive oil - 1 t	40
	Brown rice - ½ c	100
	Homemade bone broth	30
	Total	**200**
Snack	Pear, medium size	35
	Total	**35**
Dinner	Turkey burger - 4 oz raw	90
	Broccoli - ½ cup	15
	Olive oil - 1 t	40
	Total	**145**
Grand Total Day Calories		**585**

		Calories
Breakfast	Bullet Proof Coffee:	
	MCT oil - 1 T	60
	Pasture raised grass-fed butter - 1 T	110
	Organic light roast coffee - 12 oz	3
	Total	**173**
Lunch	Garbanzo stir-fry (recipe)	125
	Jasmine rice - ½ c	107
	Total	**200**
Dinner	Green garden salad:	
	Organic mixed leaves lettuce - 2 c	
	with super greens and cucumber,	
	radish, red & yellow pepper	100
	Vinaigrette - ½ T	45
	Total	**145**
Snack	Raw vegetable juice, homemade - 12 oz:	75
	Celery - 1 c	
	Red beet - ½	
	Blueberries - ¼ c	
	Ginger - ¼ t	
	Turmeric - ¼ t	
	Super greens - 2 c	
	Total	**75**
Grand Total Day Calories		**628**

		Calories
Breakfast	Oatmeal with blueberries	200
	Green tea - 20 oz	0
	Total	**200**
Lunch	Rotisserie chicken breast no skin - 3 oz	130
	Cauliflower - ½ c	15
	Brussel sprouts - ½ cup	20
	Olive oil - 1 t	40
	Total	**205**
Dinner	Homemade chicken bone broth	30
	Avocado Tuna Salad (recipe) - ½ cup:	145
	Albacore tuna	
	Avocado	
	Red apple/toasted pecans	
	Pickle juice/dried dill/cumin/salt/pepper	
	Dijon mustard	
	Total	**175**
Grand Total Day Calories		**580**

		Calories
Breakfast	Protein shake	200
	Green tea - 20 oz	0
	Total	**200**
Lunch	Chickpea, red pepper, arugula salad (recipe)	190
	Total	**190**
Dinner	Homemade chicken bone broth	30
	Mexican casserole (recipe) - ½ c	180
	Iced tea - herbal	0
	Total	**210**
Grand Total Day Calories		**600**

Triple R day questions

These are open ended questions to ask yourself on Triple R days. The intent is to help you have a critical and deep conversation with yourself. None are "yes or no" questions. There are over 100 questions here, so you can ask yourself a different question every Triple R day. Or you can ask yourself a few poignant questions at various times throughout the year on several different Triple R days.

These questions will be updated on www.2dayGift.com/Resources constantly, so keep checking.

How to use the Triple R day questions

- Read through this list and highlight the ones that stand out to you as hard questions to answer.
- On Sunday, while deciding your two Triple R days for the week, decide on the questions you want to ask yourself.
- On your Triple R day, decide on the best time to ask yourself the questions. It could be during morning meditation, at lunch instead of eating, or on a long walk when you get home. Record the conversation on your smart phone, and keep it to 10 minutes at a time.
- Occasionally listen to past answers
- Transcribe the best answers here: www.speechpad.com

General questions – that one thing

These questions are about your special talent. That thing we each do better than anyone else we know. Each of us has something. Discovering that one thing is one of the steps in developing passion. As Ben Franklin said, "if passion is our driver, let reason hold the reins." The time for reason is later.

1. What is the one thing I can do better than any person I know?
2. If I got better at that one thing, how would it make my life better?
3. If I got better at that one thing, how would that make others' lives better?
4. Why am I not doing that one thing more?

Time orientated

None of us knows how long we have left. What we do know is that it will not be long enough to accomplish everything we are capable of. We also know we waste a lot of this precious time. These questions focus your mind on priorities.

1. What would I do if I knew I had 24 hours to live?
2. What would I do if I knew I had one month to live?
3. What would I do if I knew I had one year to live?
4. What would I do if I knew I would live forever?
5. What would I do if I knew my time on earth was undermined?
6. If I was given an envelope with my exact time, place, and manner of death, would I open it?
7. What age do I feel like inside and why?

Fear orientated

These questions are about fear. Fear can seriously demotivate you. Fear can stop you in your tracks. I remember jogging in the woods and seeing a 10 foot rattlesnake stretched across the path. I changed my horizontal momentum into vertical momentum in a movement that had to be epic to watch. That was an external threat. Internal and spiritual threats are just as scary, but sometimes they are hidden. Nonetheless, they need to be examined.

1. What would I do if I was not afraid?
2. What would I do if I was always afraid?
3. Why is it possible for me to go from afraid to fearless?
4. What do I fear the most?
5. What am I most confident about?
6. What if I lost the most important item in my life?

Money orientated

Money is often misquoted as the route of all evil. For most of us, money is the tool we use to hunt and gather our food in modern times. Money may not be the root of all evil, but money can be traced as the root of bad decisions. For the first question, think of a monumental mistake you made.

1. What decision would I have made, if money wasn't an issue?
2. What would I do if I had all the riches I want?
3. What would I do if I were poor?
4. What would I do if I were rich, but knew I would lose it all tomorrow?
5. What would I do if I were rich, and I knew it would last forever?
6. IF I could only keep five possessions, what would I choose, and why?

Why me?

"Why me?" questions are about your purpose. Most people want passion and purpose in their lives, but want it handed to them. For instance you might ask, *if I were passionate about something, wouldn't I know it?* The simple answer is no; the more complicated answer would be "why not?" As with the UdP, each of us takes the path individually, even when we have a partner. As the ancient Greeks used to say "Know thyself."

1. What is my purpose?
2. Why am I so blessed?
3. Why am I so cursed?
4. Why do I take responsibility?
5. Why don't I take responsibility?
6. What do I want to do with my life?
7. What do I regret the most?
8. What am I most proud of?
9. Where will I be next year?
10. What is my story?
11. Where will I be in 10 years?
12. What do I want people to say about me at my memorial?
13. What am I good at?
14. What am I bad at?
15. What do I despise?
16. Who do I look up to?
17. What are the attributes of a real hero? How many do I have?
18. What would I change about myself? Why?
19. What do I like most about myself? Why?
20. What motivates me in my life?
21. What demotivates me?
22. How do I handle stress?
23. How do I handle depression?
24. How do I define success?
25. What are my values?
26. What am I passionate about?
27. What am I doing when I feel most like myself?
28. What was my toughest battle and how did I handle it?
29. What makes me vulnerable?
30. What makes me feel safe?
31. How am I spiritual?
32. What is in my bucket list?
33. What does "honor" mean?

34. What does "morals" mean to me?
35. How do I want to be remembered by my children, spouse, mother, father, siblings and coworkers, after I'm gone?
36. What does my ideal life look like?
37. How am I ruled by emotions?
38. How am I ruled by logic or reason?
39. What is the one thing I know for sure? How?
40. What do I doubt the most? Why?
41. What happened the last time I cried?
42. When was I hurt the most?
43. What was the hardest thing I have ever done?
44. What was the greatest day of my life?
45. What was the last miracle I saw?
46. Is there a secret no one knows about me?
47. When did I compliment a complete stranger?
48. Is there a chore I secretly like to do?
49. Am I operating on all cylinders (living to my fullest capacity)?
50. How do I deal with the "bully" within myself?
51. What am I an expert on?
52. What mistake do I keep on repeating?
53. What miracle do I refuse to believe?
54. Do I want to live in the past?
55. Am I happy?
56. What is the best compliment I ever received?
57. What is the most out-of-character decision I ever made?
58. What is my favorite book of all time?

Relationship-oriented questions

No one is an island. Even loners have to interact with other people at some time.

Warning: Theses relationship questions can be dangerous. They sound safe enough, but since most people never question their relationships, any question can make you face answers you are not prepared for. Proceed with caution. These dangerous questions are extremely important to ask.

1. What makes me a good partner?
2. What am I looking for in a life partner?
3. What is in their bucket list and how do they match with mine?
4. What kind of partner do I need to share my darkest secret with?
5. What is cheating in a relationship?
6. When was the last time I genuinely screamed at my partner?
7. If I had $5000 to spend on my partner, how would I spend it?
8. When did my partner most disappoint me?
9. When did I last disappoint my partner?
10. Why I was initially attracted to my partner?
11. How would my partner describe me?
12. How would I write the perfect love note?
13. How would I compliment my spouse?
14. What will I miss about my partner when he/she is gone?
15. What will they miss about me when I'm gone?
16. What would my partner and I do if he/she had one month to live?
17. What would my partner and I do if I had one month to live?
18. How would our relationship change if we both lived forever?
19. Are we happy?
20. Do we want to continue as we lived in the past?

Societal questions

Where do I fit in society? I find these the least important, but once you "know thyself" and you know your partner, you will want to consider how you fit into the world at large. These questions might have been answered before, but now the focus is on you and the world. As my dad use to shout every morning on the front porch of my childhood home, "**Hello World!**"

1. Do I have an obligation to society?
2. Does charity work?
3. Would I accept charity for myself? My family?
4. What is government's role in my life?
5. What is the spiritual world's role in my life?
6. Have I ever met someone truly evil?
7. Have I ever met someone truly good?
8. When was the last time I was kind to a stranger?
9. Am I entitled to anything?
10. What does my God look like?
11. When is it ever acceptable to lie?
12. What would I give up to be safe from terrorism?

Sample journal pages

The following pages can be photocopied and used for journaling. Use Christie's journal in chapter 8 for an example of how to fill them out.

For a template you can fill out on your computer or mobile device, go to www.2dayGift.com/resources

UdP
2 DAY GIFT OF WELLNESS

Day ______________________

Date ______________________

☐ Triple R (2x/week) Total calories = 600 max

Weight ____________ Slept ______________________

Steps ____________ Hours of Calorie Reduction ______________

	Food	Calories (Triple R days only, 600 max)
Breakfast		
Snack		
Lunch		
Snack		
Dinner		

Notes

UdP
2 DAY GIFT OF WELLNESS

Christie's journal weeks 2–8

Christie's journals are continued here from chapter 8. These excerpts represent her actual comments and her advancement from weeks 2–8. I listed her Triple R days, weights and comments. As her mentor, I listed my comments as well.

Week 2

Tuesday – Triple R day

Thursday – Triple R day

Weight: 207.2

Week 2 Notes:

Feeling much better today. Got some sleep. Found myself not feeling hungry at all. It felt great! Getting sleep really does help uplift my overall sense of wellbeing. Ended up having 1 bite of the dinner I prepared for my son, Chicken Alfredo. I know it put me over the 600 calories but not sure how much. I would guess 50 calories. I'm not going to beat myself up over it. I am just learning about myself and my patterns. It's much easier when Dylan's not here. And it wasn't even because I was hungry. Trying to be completely honest in these journals as I feel I would be only cheating myself if I omit things.

Feeling good today. This week's Triple R days seem much easier than last week's.

I had a conversation with my son which could have been very stressful but I managed to stay calm and not get as upset as I normally would. I couldn't push it off as there had been resentment building on both our parts and the timing just happened to work out for us, although it was totally unplanned.

Since the conversation ended up taking quite a while, I decided to leave the dishes for the next day, something I would normally not do because seeing dishes in the sink in the morning stresses me out, but not this time. I was totally okay with it.

As for the "couples" issues, I think the only reason my husband and I are doing the Triple R days on the same day is that my husband usually prepares our morning protein shake while I am getting ready for work and on these days, it is made differently as the peanut butter is omitted.

We don't eat the same things at all. I usually cook my food and Dylan's food because for the most part, we eat the same proteins. I eat veggies and the boys really don't. Other than that we are both trying to be supportive of each other but our process is very different. I meditate and journal, and my husband doesn't. I love silence, but my husband not so much so although we are doing this together, it is a very separate journey in many ways.

Dr. Michael's [founder mentor] comments:

Christie, you are doing very well. Your journaling is very detailed. Let me know what you are doing for the REST on Triple R day. That is the most difficult. As you will notice the Reduce part of the Triple R gets easier. Although weight loss is not a goal, you have lost an average of ⅓ lb per DAY, since you started. This is an indication that your body is responding. I know it is frustrating to see weight fluctuate throughout the week, but use the lowest weight because that is the closest to your truest weight (without changes of water weight). Keep up the good work. 4.6 lbs, wow!

Week 2 Reflections

Week #2 seemed to go much more smoothly. My mind, as well as my body, are starting to get used to the routine. I find myself looking forward to the Triple R days, mostly the relaxation part. The food prep is still quite a task but I suspect it will get easier. I'm not worrying about the weight loss as much either.

I went to breakfast with a friend who came up last night. Felt like I still managed to be mindful about what I was eating.

Dr. Michael:

Christie, you are a rock star. I think you are doing well, pushing things until tomorrow that can be pushed, without guilt. I understand about your conversation with your son. Conversations with significant people, even when not controversial, are critical conversations, so it is difficult to put them off. I think you discovered that if you push off non-vital events (dishes) you have more patience for the critical events. I thank you for sharing that story.

You mention your food prep is a daunting task. Maybe reflect on some easy, standard, Triple R day meals. It's two days a week, so try not to make them any more difficult than necessary. Mine are simple compared to yours. Yesterday I had:

2 eggs for breakfast	140
1 can of crab meat with pickles and mustard	80
2 more eggs throughout the day	140
Very small steak (3 oz.)	156
Small piece of broiled halibut (3oz)	108
	Total 624
	(a little over)

Admittedly this is a lot of protein and no vegetables, but I was on an international trip and had limited choices. The point is to try to make it simple for these days.

The goal is to give your system a pause, a rest, while not stressing it out by being hungry.

The bottom line is, you and your husband are doing great. The amount of detail you provide is outstanding. Keep it up!!

Christie's response:

Dr. Michael, thanks for the feedback! As for meal prep, I think right now it is difficult because I love cooking, especially for my son, but because of Triple R days, I end up making a couple of different meals, sometimes up to 3 the night before a Triple R day. He will be going back to school in a few weeks and I think that will make it easier.

Eggs are so easy, I absolutely love them but unfortunately I am allergic to them. I have been buying rotisserie chicken as the "easy" protein to use on Triple R days. So far I love this whole process so I plan on keeping it up.

Journal Week #3

Monday – Triple R day

Weight: 206.2

Notes

My husband is out of town with his daughter and they will be back Wednesday night so I switched up my Triple R days. Today I did not feel hungry at all. Was going to run some errands after work but thought about how I should be respecting the Triple R so instead I came straight home. My son was home with some friends watching baseball. I made them some appetizers while sipping on my bone broth. I came upstairs to relax and do some reading and journaling as I answered one of the Triple R questions. I meditate and journal every morning. Very relaxing day. Best Triple R day so far!

Wednesday – Triple R day

Notes

I went over my calorie content today. My husband's daughter is visiting from AZ so once again I prepared a couple of different meals tonight but I realize this is completely my choice. I ended up tasting the pasta bake, which accounted for the extra calories. Still feeling great though!

Dr. Michael:

You are doing so great. You got this Triple R day down. The rest of your days are also healthy! I am very proud of you and your progress! Best Triple R day EVER! Look at your weight drop. You are really controlling the stress on your Triple R day and you are meditating almost every day. WAY to GO!

Christie's response:

Thanks Mike! I am very excited! Things are progressing and although I realize I will have good days and bad days, I know now that I don't have to beat myself up about the bad ones, just keep plugging away. Hope to get back to working out next week. I love the walks but not when it is 110 outside. Also, on my Triple R days I would love to do some gentle yoga.

For the record, I have not missed a day of meditating since January 1st :) First time in years that this has been the case and I am very happy about this. Longest I have gone continuously was to get to May and then something happens and I start skipping it. Same with journaling. Also, I am loving the Triple R questions. Very thought provoking!

Week 3 Notes

Today was more stressful than planned. But I feel that having a couple of weeks of Triple R "mentality" under my belt is really helping me handle life much better overall. I also agree with you Mike, that journaling my food/experiences every day is key for me to stay on track.

Rough day. My husband and I went to the movies and lunch to celebrate our anniversary, which is tomorrow. Felt like it was a good day until we ended up at the casino, where we lost a bunch of money and I didn't get to eat. Did not drink alcohol though. On the way home my husband stopped at McDonald's and got an ice cream cone, some fries, then came home and made some hotdogs. I chose to not have any of that. I feel like I am still trying to eat mindfully and make healthy choices. Or if I splurge on one meal, I balance it out with the next. That part all feels good. Overall mood for the end of the day: not great.

Week 3 Reflections

Overall, I felt it was a good week although I was a little disappointed on how it ended. My weight went up for a couple of days, but with the wine and salty food I consumed I am not worried about it. Felt like I did better than I have in the past when there is company here. I didn't go all out although I notice that when I drink alcohol, I feel more like munching on some "not as healthy" food choices. Also, I am finding that red wine causes my feet and ankles to swell, probably along with the salty foods. I saw my weight fluctuate but at least it is moving in the right direction. All in all, still feeling great.

Dr. Michael:

I noticed you have been eating a lot of pizza and popcorn. These two foods make me put on a lot of water weight. It also seems to take a while to lose that weight, but have faith, your true weight is probably a few pounds less than you think. I can tell you are getting fitter and healthier by your comments.

If you only lost a pound a week and kept it off, in 6 months you would be 22 lbs lighter. On any other diet you would have lost the

10-15 lbs and already put it back on. You are probably losing more like 1.5 lbs/week, but I bet you can feel the difference in the way your clothes feel.

You mentioned some foods and red wine make your ankles swell. This might be due to a micro allergy of some food or food combinations you are eating.

If you are feeling discouraged and want to increase your weight loss, research shows a high protein diet is the fastest way. But I would discourage that in your case, because you seem to be focused on a healthy and balanced diet, which probably will bring longer term success.

The bottom line is that I think you are doing great. Your true weight loss for the three weeks is probably 5-6 lbs. I'd cut back on the high carb snacks if you want to see the scale show your true weight. Keep up the good work.

You're doing fantastic!!

Christie's response:

Thanks for the feedback Mike. Some very good suggestions. I have had a food allergy test before and try to avoid anything that may trigger allergies. With that being said, I occasionally eat eggs and gluten and that could cause some inflammation. The pizza crust is gluten free, so that is better than eating regular crust. I am beginning to suspect there is something going on with the red wine. I have another allergy test at the end of the month so maybe we can find out what may be causing it.

Journal Week #4

Tuesday – Triple R day

Notes

Feeling just okay today. Took advantage of the Triple R day, came from work and took a nap. Pushed out my errands till tomorrow. Learning to respect the Triple R. A bit hungry today but it wasn't too bad.

Thursday – Triple R day

Week 4 Notes

Weight: 206.2

Happy with the weight number for the last two days. Feeling good, except for the hives, they are getting worse. Again, put off errands. Went out in the backyard and read a book. Haven't done that in a long time. It felt wonderful!

Week 4 Reflections

Woke up one day to a weight gain I wasn't expecting. Felt a bit discouraged, but healthier so I guess that is a good thing. Still committed to making healthy food choices, mindful eating.

Met up with some friends for wine tasting and lunch. Expected my weight to jump due to the alcohol and salt from the fries and pizza, but I am not worried now as I know this is my lifestyle and I can have days like this, combined with my Triple R days and other regular days of mindful eating. I am feeling pretty good.

I am totally fine with my fun day out celebrating. I also found that it was very easy to stay committed to a day of mindful eating after yesterday when in the past I may not have. Feelings of guilt can wreak havoc on staying committed to a healthy lifestyle.

Now I'm beginning to look forward to Triple R days.

I feel like I am finally getting into a routine that is working for me. It is getting easier to commit to Triple R days, to allowing myself fun, celebratory days and to stay focused on the other days. I was pleased with my week overall. As I said in my notes for Sunday evening, when I beat myself up over "slipping" or not seeing results on the scale, it can really cause the very stress that I am trying to address on Triple R days, and for that matter, every day. Guilt and shame are emotions that can sabotage my efforts to stay committed to a healthy lifestyle

Dr. Michael:

Great job on journaling. 7 lbs is pretty good! Weight fluctuations happen if you don't follow a specific diet (like Atkins or Paleo). The daily weight goes up and down. But your weight loss is real. It can be frustrating, but weight is a data point and a by-product of your healthy living. That will make your weight loss sustainable. Congrats!

Journal Week #5 (begin 2nd month)

Weight: 203.2

Tuesday – Triple R day

Slept: 7.5 hours

Physical Activity: None

Hours/Calorie Red 9:30pm – 9:00am 2.5+24+9.0 = 35.5

Notes

Feeling good today. I was talking to a friend about how having a Triple R day forces me to take time for myself, to slow down. I don't think I would be making "me time" a priority if it wasn't for this program. Very happy I found it!

Thursday – Triple R day

Slept: 14.5 hours

Physical Activity: None

Hours/Calorie Red 12:00am – 11:30am 24+11.5 = 35.5

Notes

Very rough day today in regards to stress. Went to bed at 7:30pm

Week 5 Notes

Today I was mindful that I allowed myself to cut loose a bit. With the stress of the week, I am okay with it. Our son, who is causing some of the stress, is leaving tomorrow so I will be back on track. Again, it's a lifestyle that I am happily committed to now.

Dr. Michael:

Another stellar week, Christie. I'm going through all the logs and noticed that you have lost 8.8 lbs in 5 weeks or 2.2 lbs a week – very impressive.

Christie's response:

Thanks, Dr. Michael! I feel fortunate that I get this opportunity. It came at the perfect time.

Week 5 Reflection

Dealing with some very stressful family issues but still trying to stay focused on my health. Went to bed early last night so as not to eat or drink alcohol.

The end of a long stressful weekend so I indulged a bit. Back to it tomorrow. On a good note, I didn't finish off the bottle of wine, which is something I would have done in the past.

Dr. Michael:

Christie, great job on the journaling and congratulations on your weight loss. You are really doing well. I hope your family issues can be resolved enough to decrease your stress. The extra sleep is beneficial and I hope you can use your Triple R day techniques on your regular days to help with the stress.

Christie's response:

We went out to happy hour last night and both of us realized we could not eat as much as we normally would. We went to the movies afterward and the same thing went for the popcorn. In fact, my husband threw away what was left of the large, when there was still a FREE refill for it. I think this is the first time I can ever remember him doing this (unless it was really bad popcorn, but this was one he likes). Slowly but surely, habits are changing!

Well to say that this was a stressful week would be putting it mildly. All in all, I was very proud of the way I handled it for the most part. Thursday night, instead of reaching for food or wine, I just went to bed. I can't remember the last time I went to bed so early.

I respected the Triple R, which is saying I respected myself. The weekend I was a bit looser with my eating but now that our son is gone, I expect things to be much better in many different ways. I won't be cooking meals for him that I am tempted to eat. I won't feel guilty for coming upstairs to meditate and journal. Taking time for me is much easier when he is not here.

We will be traveling to AZ this coming weekend so I will be sticking to my Triple R days Tuesday and Thursday of this week. Again, with being in a routine, I think it will be easier to not go too far off the rails. I have been feeling so much better in regards to doing something for my health. Being able to see the effect is really helpful in motivating me to keep doing what I am doing.

Journal Week #6

Tuesday – Triple R day

Weight: 206.0

Slept: 7.5 hours

Physical Activity: None

Hours/Calorie Red 10:00pm – 9:00am 2+24+9.0 = 35.0

Notes

Feeling okay today. Came home and took a nap. Things are still a little wonky in regards to the stress going on but I am trying to manage it with the tools I have along with the UdP process, which I think is helping.

Feeling a little better today. The Deepak 21 day meditation I am doing is helping as well as the journaling. Reducing stress is the key.

Thursday – Triple R day

Slept: 5.5 hours

Physical Activity: None

Hours/Calorie Red 12:00 am – 11:00 am 24+11.0 = 35.0

Notes

Indulged a bit last night so was happy to see my weight did not go up too much this morning. Traveling on a Triple R day but it hasn't been bad. Driving to AZ so I don't need to eat tonight on the way.

Week 6 Notes

I still feeling like I am practicing mindful eating as we went out for Italian food at lunch. I chose a salad knowing we were having pasta for dinner. I also cut back on alcohol after a few drinks.

Feeling like I am veering off track a bit but didn't drink as much as I normally would. Lack of sleep is catching up to me and it makes it hard to make smart choices. Even though I am showing a decent amount of sleep hours, I am not sleeping well. I wake up several times a night.

Felt good about my choices in lunch and dinner since they were both at fast food restaurants. I did find myself snacking last night as we sat around drinking and socializing.

Week 6 Reflection

I found that being on vacation definitely makes it harder to stay on track. I felt like I did okay, meaning could have done better, could have done worse. Wasn't able to weigh myself and I feel that could have helped. I am looking forward to being back home tomorrow and a Triple R day on Tuesday.

Journal Week #7

Weight: 202.6

Tuesday – Triple R day

Slept: 7 hours

Physical Activity: None

Hours/Calorie Red 8pm – 9:00am 4+24+9 = 37.0

Thursday – Triple R day

Slept: 8.5 hours

Physical Activity: None

Hours/Calorie Red 8:30pm – 11:30am 3.5+24+11.5 = 39

Notes

So happy to see the weight number this morning! For me, it validated that I am on the right path, committed to my overall health and that this program is sustainable.

Dr. Michael:

Great job, as usual Christie. It is pretty exciting to go on vacation and not get totally off track. Proud of you.

Friday – Regular Day

Slept: 9 hours

Physical Activity: None

Notes

It felt great seeing the number on the scale this morning. Inspired to keep going! I also seem to be handling stress better. Car broke down today, my husband is out of town yet I managed to go outside with a glass of wine and read my book and not stress about it.

Saturday – Regular Day

Weight: 202.6

Slept: 10 hours

Physical Activity: None

Notes

Good day today. I realized that my tolerance for alcohol has gone way down. I can't drink as much as I used to, which isn't a bad thing.

Sunday – Regular Day

Weight: 202.6

Slept: 10 hours

Physical Activity: None

Notes

Looking forward to getting back on track – Triple R day tomorrow!

Didn't realize I didn't write any notes this night. Let's just go with that it was good day. Was happy with my weight this morning after the weekend. From Monday to Monday there was no weight gain. It seems to be getting easier. Not feeling as hungry.

Weight: 201.6 – Yay! Lowest weight since I can remember – back in 2012?

Reflection

Felt like I had a really good week. Back on track after being on vacation. Weight loss still going in the right direction and I am very pleased with that. Feeling really good and loving the process.

Journal Week #8

Monday – Regular Day

Weight: 204.4

Slept: 7 hours

Physical Activity: None

Notes

Not feeling well today, emotionally and physically. I think the Mexican casserole upset my stomach last night and today. Had another doctor's appointment today for more allergy testing. Still breaking out in hives and today it just got to me, plus I did not get a good night's sleep last night so I am tired, which always causes me to be more emotional.

Tuesday – Triple R day

Weight: 203.2

Slept: 8 hours

Physical Activity: None

Hours/Calorie Red 7:30pm – 9:00am 4.5+24+9 = 37.0

Notes

I wasn't feeling well today but more due to lack of sleep. Had an appointment this afternoon but cancelled it so I could come home and sleep. Was able to get a couple of hours of sleep, but that was it. I will take what I can get. Feeling better physically. Triple R day today went well.

Wednesday – Regular Day

Weight: 201.8

Slept: 8.5 hours

Physical Activity: None

Notes

Was very happy to see the number on the scale this morning. It also felt good to get some sleep. Still feeling very good about the program!

Dr. Michael:

Interesting to note how your weight spiked 3 lbs when you ate the Mexican casserole. Was your body telling you to stop that? Glad you didn't get frustrated. You're doing great!

Christie's response:

Wow, I hadn't even realized that. That is very interesting. Luckily I didn't have to eat any more, my husband took care of the rest, haha.

Thursday – Triple R day

Weight: 202

Slept: 8.5 hours

Physical Activity: None

Hours/Calorie Red 10:30pm – 11am 1.5+24+11 = 36.5

Notes

Feeling good, just a little hungry today. Lots going on so I tried to get in a little bit of relaxation by getting a pedicure. Unfortunately I had to answer panic texts from son, who of course needed me to take care of something immediately. Darn kids

Friday – Regular Day

Weight: 200.2 – Woohoo! Lowest weight in at least 4 years

Slept: 10.5 hours

Physical Activity: None

Notes

Good day today. I splurged a bit but will be back on track tomorrow. Drank some wine and the good news is I don't feel like drinking as much as I used to.

Saturday – Regular Day

Weight: 201.8

Slept: 9.5 hours

Physical Activity: None

Notes

A day of home improvements, painting, so a very good, productive day. Feeling good. Chose to make healthy food rather than fast food. I took a couple of breaks to make the food so I didn't get hungry and snack on junk.

Week 8 Reflections

It's been a fairly good week. Saw my lowest weight in over 4 years and I was very happy about that.

I think because I have several weeks of the UdP under my belt, it was easier to make smarter food choices. When you are working 10+ hours a day on manual projects, sometimes it is easier to grab fast food or junk food but I was motivated by my weight loss this week to take time out to make some healthy food. Looking forward to what next week brings as far as the number on the scale.

I did get a pedicure on one of my Triple R days last week but my meditation and journaling have been slipping. Need to get back on that.

Dr. Michael:

Christie, sorry you are having so much stress and emotions this week. It's so easy to give up on healthy eating and rejuvenating when life hands you a rotten deal. But, now is exactly the time to try to put off the stress for a couple of days. I don't know what the issue is, so I might be talking out of turn, but usually situations that upset us also take a long time to resolve. So a few days of letting go of the problem won't make a difference in the long run but will add years to your life with the 2 day break. I know it's hard, and I wish you the best possible outcome.

Christie's response:

Mike, thanks for the kind words. I honestly believe if I didn't have the UdP process in place, I might have gone totally off the rails. The fact that I do has helped me tremendously.

I woke up Friday morning and had a good number on the scale and that made me feel good. We met up with some good friends for a quick visit and I had a salad for lunch. My husband and I were going to go to the movies and instead of eating out beforehand, I cooked something relatively healthy. I still allowed myself some popcorn and frozen yogurt afterwards and then decided against any alcohol tonight, which means I don't go all out, instead choosing one or two "not as healthy" choices rather than all of them.

The next couple of days I will eat healthy. Monday is my birthday so I may splurge a bit and then Tuesday is another Triple R day. I am much more in tune as well with how certain foods are affecting me, and which ones are causing me to retain water and swell up.

I told my husband today that this is now my lifestyle. I look forward to the Triple R days rather than dread them. They give me an opportunity to nurture myself (emotionally/spiritually/physically) and that is a good thing. Hope to get back to meditating and journaling Monday.

Reflections

This has been a very tough week for me emotionally. As I said in response to your comments, Mike, I think that if I didn't have the UdP process in place, it could have been worse. I am so close to being under 200, I have my eye on the carrot so to speak and it keeps me motivated. I am very grateful for this process and for all I am learning.

Dr. Michael:

Christie, I'm the same way, very close (and occasionally touching) a number I hadn't seen in 15 years. But the worry and the anxiety about weight is counter-productive. Just keep on trucking. You are still doing great.

Christie's response:

I agree Mike. Focusing on goals causes me to lose sight of what I am actually trying to do, which is have a healthy lifestyle which includes learning to deal with everyday stress in a healthy manner. If I get too focused on the number on the scale, I totally agree it is counterproductive in that it causes the very stress I am trying to reduce. Thank you for your words of encouragement and your support!

Further reflections

The UdP process is becoming second nature to me and I find myself looking forward to the Triple R days. Weight loss is slow but I am choosing not to focus on that. I am choosing to focus instead on how I am feeling and what I am learning about the reasons I overeat, and why I eat food that is not good for me. Good stuff!

I have been under a lot of stress and consider it a win that I am not gaining weight. Being aware of my behavior is the first step in changing it.

Another good day even with the number on the scale. I know it was high because last night I overindulged a bit with a few drinks and some salty snacks. Back on track today. Boy, do I look forward to Triple R days!

My clothes are feeling much looser. Since the beginning of the year I am down 14 pounds which for me is huge since I haven't been able to lose weight for years.

Maybe it was because I wasn't so committed or hadn't found something that appealed to me. I feel like I have finally found it!

As long as it keeps going in the right direction, I know I am doing what I need to do to get healthy. It's all about a healthy lifestyle.

Dr. Michael:

Amen. Stress is hard. Losing weight while stressed doesn't work for most people. The fact that you haven't gained shows your previous weight loss is sustainable. Excellent.

"The UdP addresses the whole mind/body/ spirit connection, which is something that really resonates with me." -Christie Z, California

---

Chapter Sources

Sources for Introduction

Aamodt, S. (May 2016). Why you can't lose weight on a diet: The problem isn't willpower. It's neuroscience. *New York Times,* Op Ed, SR1.

Fothergill, E. Gau, J., Howard, L., Kerns, J., Knuth, N., Brychta, R., Chen, K., Skarulis, M., ... Hall, K. (March 2016). Persistent metabolic adaptation six years after "The Biggest Loser" competition. *Obesity*, 1-8. doi:10.1002/oby.21538

Lucan, S. C., & DiNicolantonio, J. J. (2015). How calorie-focused thinking about obesity and related diseases may mislead and harm public health; An alternative. *Public Health Nutrition, 18*(4), 571-581. doi:http://dx.doi.org/10.1017/S1368980014002559

Monteiro, C. A., & Cannon, G. (2015). Calories do not add up. *Public Health Nutrition, 18*(4), 569-570. doi:http://dx.doi.org/10.1017/S1368980015000014

Pekkarinen, T., Kaukua, J., & Mustajoki, P. (2015). Long-term weight maintenance after a 17-week weight loss intervention with or without a one-year maintenance program: A randomized controlled trial. *Journal of Obesity,* doi:http://dx.doi.org/10.1155/2015/651460

Pontzer, H., Raichlen, D. A., Wood, B. M., Mabulla, A. P., Racette, S. B., & Marlowe, F. W. (2012). Hunter-gatherer energetics and human obesity. *Plos One*, 7(7), e40503. doi:10.1371/journal.pone.0040503

Rosenbaum, M., Hirsch, J., Gallagher, D. A., & Leibel, R. L. (2008). Long-term persistence of adaptive thermogenesis in subjects who have maintained a reduced body weight. *The American Journal Of Clinical Nutrition*, 88(4), 906-912.

Sources for Chapter 1

Aamodt, S. (May 2016). Why you can't lose weight on a diet: The problem isn't willpower. It's neuroscience. *New York Times*, Op Ed, SR1.

Fothergill, E. Gau, J., Howard, L., Kerns, J., Knuth, N., Brychta, R., Chen, K., Skarulis, M., ... Hall, K. (March 2016). Persistent metabolic adaptation six years after "The Biggest Loser" competition. *Obesity*, 1-8. doi:10.1002/oby.21538

Hopkins, M., Gibbons, C., Caudwell, P., Hellström, P. M., Näslund, E., King, N. A., & Blundell, J. E. (2014). The adaptive metabolic response to exercise-induced weight loss influences both energy expenditure and energy intake. *European Journal of Clinical Nutrition, 68*(5), 581-6. doi:http://dx.doi.org/10.1038/ejcn.2013.277

Lucan, S. C., & DiNicolantonio, J. J. (2015). How calorie-focused thinking about obesity and related diseases may mislead and harm public health: An alternative. *Public Health Nutrition, 18*(4), 571-581. doi:http://dx.doi.org/10.1017/S1368980014002559

Neel J.V., Weder, A.B., & Julius S. (1998). Type II diabetes, essential hypertension, and obesity as "syndromes of impaired genetic homeostasis": the "thrifty genotype" hypothesis enters the 21st century. *Perspect. Biol. Med.*, 42(1), 44-74.

Dulloo, A. G., & Montani, J. (2015). Pathways from dieting to weight regain, to obesity and to the metabolic syndrome: an overview. *Obesity Reviews*, 161-176. doi:10.1111/obr.12250

Pontzer, H., Raichlen, D. A., Wood, B. M., Mabulla, A. P., Racette, S. B., & Marlowe, F. W. (2012). Hunter-gatherer energetics and human obesity. *Plos One*, 7(7), doi:e40503. doi:10.1371/journal.pone.0040503

Sources for Chapter 2

Aamodt, S. (May 2016). Why you can't lose weight on a diet: The problem isn't willpower. It's neuroscience. *New York Times*, Op Ed, SR1.

Fothergill E. Gau, J., Howard, L., Kerns, J., Knuth, N., Brychta, R., Chen, K., Skarulis, M., ... Hall, K. (March 2016). Persistent metabolic adaptation six years after "The Biggest Loser" competition. *Obesity,* 1-8. doi:10.1002/oby.21538

Neel J.V., Weder, A.B., & Julius S. (1998). Type II diabetes, essential hypertension, and obesity as "syndromes of impaired genetic homeostasis": the "thrifty genotype" hypothesis enters the 21st century. *Perspect. Biol. Med.*; 42(1), 44-74.

Pontzer, H. (July 2015). Constrained total energy expenditure and the evolutionary biology of energy balance. *Exercise and Sport Sciences Reviews*, 43 (3), 110-116.

Sources for Chapter 3

Anton, S. & Leeuwenburgh, C., (2013). Fasting or caloric restriction for healthy aging. *Experimental Gerontology;* 48, 1003–1005.

Bouchonville, M., Armamento-Villareal, R., Shah, K., Napoli, N., Sinacore, D. R., Qualls, C., & Villareal, D. T. (2014). Weight loss, exercise or both and cardiometabolic risk factors in obese older adults: Results of a randomized controlled trial. *International Journal of Obesity, 38*(3), 423-31. doi:http://dx.doi.org/10.1038/ijo.2013.122

Kluever Romo, L., & Dailey, R. M. (2014). Weighty dynamics: Exploring couples' perceptions of post-weight loss interaction. *Health Communication*, 29(2), 193-204. doi:10.1080/10410236.2012.736467

Jackson, S. E., Steptoe, A., & Wardle, J. (2015). The influence of partner's behavior on health behavior change: the English Longitudinal Study of Ageing. *JAMA Internal Medicine*, 175(3), 385-392. doi:10.1001/jamainternmed.2014.7554

Mousavi, S., Rezaei, S., Bagnhi, S. (Spring 2014). Effect of fasting on mental health in the general population of Kermanshah, Iran. *Journal of Fasting and Health*; (2)2, 65-70.

Rohner-Jeanrenaud, F., Noquerias, R. (2015). Endocrine control of energy homeostasis. *Molecular and Cellular Endocrinology*, 418(4), 1-2.

Stelter, R. (2015). "I tried so many diets, now I want to do it differently" A single case study on coaching for weight loss. *International Journal of Qualitative Studies on Health and wellbeing, 10.* doi:http://dx.doi.org/10.3402/qhw.v10.26925

Waldo, O. A. (2015). The 3 "rs"--relax, reflect, and regroup. *Journal of the American College of Cardiology, 66*(11), 1303-1306. doi:http://dx.doi.org/10.1016/j.jacc.2015.07.054

Sources for Chapter 4

Fothergill, E. Gau, J., Howard, L., Kerns, J., Knuth, N., Brychta, R., Chen, K., Skarulis, M., ... Hall, K. (March 2016). Persistent metabolic adaptation six years after "The Biggest Loser" competition. *Obesity*, 1-8. doi:10.1002/oby.21538

Pekkarinen, T., Kaukua, J., & Mustajoki, P. (2015). Long-term weight maintenance after a 17-week weight loss intervention with or without a one-year maintenance program: A randomized controlled trial. *Journal of Obesity.* doi:http://dx.doi.org/10.1155/2015/651460

Rosenbaum, M., Hirsch, J., Gallagher, D. A., & Leibel, R. L. (2008). Long-term persistence of adaptive thermogenesis in subjects who have maintained a reduced body weight. *The American Journal Of Clinical Nutrition*, 88(4), 906-912.

Sources for Chapter 5

Chowdhury, E. A., Richardson, J. D., Tsintzas, K., Thompson, D., & Betts, J. A. (2016). Effect of extended morning fasting upon ad libitum lunch intake and associated metabolic and hormonal responses in obese adults. *International Journal of Obesity, 40*(2), 305-311. doi:http://dx.doi.org/10.1038/ijo.2015.154

Ho, S., Wu, Y., Chen, Y., & Yang, S. (2014). The effects of feeding time and time-restricted feeding on the fattening traits of white roman geese. *Animal: An International Journal of Animal Bioscience, 8*(3), 395-400. doi:http://dx.doi.org/10.1017/S1751731113002383

Riera-Crichton, D. & Tefft, N. (2014). Macronutrients and obesity: Revisiting the calories in, calories out framework. *Economics & Human Biology, 14, 33-49.* doi:10.1016/j.ehb.2014.04.002

Sources for Chapter 7

Aamodt, S. (May 2016). Why you can't lose weight on a diet: The problem isn't willpower. It's neuroscience. *New York Times*, Op Ed, SR1.

Anton, S. & Leeuwenburgh, C., (2013). Fasting or caloric restriction for healthy aging. *Experimental Gerontology;* 48(2013), 1003–1005.

Bonorden, M. L., Rogozina, O. P., Kluczny, C. M., Grossmann, M. E., Grambsch, P. L., Grande, J. P., & ... Cleary, M. P. (2009). Intermittent Calorie Restriction Delays Prostate Tumor Detection and Increases Survival Time in TRAMP Mice. *Nutrition & Cancer*, 61(2), 265-275. doi:10.1080/01635580802419798

Christensen, M. (2014). *Kunlun System: The path of inner alchemy leading to the truth within*. Primordial Alchemist

Covey, S. *(1989). Seven habits of highly effective people: Restoring the character ethic*. Simon and Schuster, New York.

Hoddy, K., Kroeger, C., Trepanowski, J., Barnosky, A., Bhutani, S., & Varady, K. (2015). Safety of alternate day fasting and effect on disordered eating behaviors. *Nutrition Journal;* 14-44. DOI 10.1186/s12937-015-0029-9

Lyer, P. (Nov 2014). The art of stillness. *TedTalk*. Retrived from https://www.ted.com/talks/pico_iyer_the_art_of_stillness?

Mousavi, S., Rezaei, S., Bagnhi, S. (Spring 2014). Effect of fasting on mental health in the general population of Kermanshah, Iran. *Journal of Fasting and Health*; (2) 2: 65-70.

Ordonez, L., Schweitzer, M., Galinsky, A., & Baserman, M. (Febuary 2009). Goals gone wild: The systematic side effects of overprescribing goal setting. *Academy of Management Perspectives; (43):1,* 6 - 16.

Rohner-Jeanrenaud, F., Noquerias, R. (2015). Endocrine control of energy homeostasis. *Molecular and Cellular Endocrinology*, (418) 4:1-2.

Sato, W., Kochiyama, T., Uono, S., Kubota, Y., Sawada, R., Yoshimura S., & Toichi, M. (2015). The structural neural substrate of subjective happiness. *Scientific Reports* 5, Article number: 16891.

Sources for Chapter 9

Berry, D. C., Schwartz, T. A., McMurray, R. G., Skelly, A. H., Neal, M., Hall, E. G., & Melkus, G. (2014). The family partners for health study: A cluster randomized controlled trial for child and parent weight management. *Nutrition & Diabetes, 4* - 9. doi:http://dx.doi.org/10.1038/nutd.2013.42

Dulloo, A. G., & Montani, J. (2015). Pathways from dieting to weight regain, to obesity and to the metabolic syndrome: an overview. *Obesity Reviews*, 161-176. doi:10.1111/obr.12250

Hansen, N. V., Brændgaard, P., Hjørnholm, C., & La Cour, S. (2014). Qualitative research building real-life interventions: User-involving development of a mindfulness-based lifestyle change support program for overweight citizens. *European Journal of Clinical Nutrition, 68*(10), 1129-33. doi:http://dx.doi.org/10.1038/ejcn.2014.106

Jackson, S. E., Steptoe, A., & Wardle, J. (2015). The influence of partner's behavior on health behavior change: the English Longitudinal Study of Ageing. *JAMA Internal Medicine*, 175(3), 385-392. doi:10.1001/jamainternmed.2014.7554

Kushner, R. F. (2008). Companion dogs as weight loss partners. *Obesity Management, 4* (5), 232-235. doi:http://dx.doi.org/10.1089/obe.2008.0225

MacLean, P.S., Higgins, J.A., Giles E.D., Sherk V.D., & Jackman M.R. (2015). The role for adipose tissue in weight regain after weight loss. *Obesity Review*. 16(Suppl. 1), 45–54.

Pressfield, S.(2002). *The war of art: Winning the inner creative battle.* Rugged Land, New York.

Stelter, R. (2015). "I tried so many diets, now I want to do it differently." A single case study on coaching for weight loss. *International Journal of Qualitative Studies on Health and Wellbeing, 10.* doi:http://dx.doi.org/10.3402/qhw.v10.26925

Theiss, J. A., Carpenter, A. M. & Leustek, J. (2016). Partner facilitation an partner interference in individuals' weight loss goals. *Qualitative Health Research*, 26 (10),1318-1330. DOI: 10.1177/1049732315583980

Wolever, R. Q., Simmons, L. A., Sforzo, G. A., Dill, D., Kaye, M., Bechard, E. M., et al. (2013). A systematic review of the literature on health and wellness coaching: Defining a key behavioral intervention in Healthcare. *Global Advances in Health and Medicine*, 2(4), 38-57.

Sources for Chapter 10

Bouchonville, M., Armamento-villareal, R., Shah, K., Napoli, N., Sinacore, D. R., Qualls, C., & Villareal, D. T. (2014). Weight loss, exercise. or both and cardiometabolic risk factors in obese older adults: Results of a randomized controlled trial. *International Journal of Obesity, 38*(3), 423-31. doi:http://dx.doi.org/10.1038/ijo.2013.122

Clark, J. E, (Apr 2015). Diet, exercise or diet with exercise: comparing the effectiveness of treatment options for weight loss and changes in fitness for adults (18-65 years old) who are overfat, or obese; systematic review and meta-analysis. *Journal of Diabetes & Metabolic Disorders*, 14, 1-46.

Hopkins, M., Gibbons, C., Caudwell, P., Hellström, P. M., Näslund, E., King, N. A., & Blundell, J. E. (2014). The adaptive metabolic response to exercise-induced weight loss influences both energy expenditure and energy intake. *European Journal of Clinical Nutrition, 68*(5), 581-6. doi: http://dx.doi.org/10.1038/ejcn.2013.277

Kong Z, Fan X, Sun S, Song L, Shi Q, & Nie J (2016). Comparison of high-intensity interval training and moderate-to-vigorous continuous training for cardio-metabolic health and exercise enjoyment in obese young women: A randomized controlled trial. *PLoS ONE*, 11(7), e0158589. doi:10.1371/journal.pone.0158589

Lucan, S. C., & DiNicolantonio, J. J. (2015). How calorie-focused thinking about obesity and related diseases may mislead and harm public health: An alternative. *Public Health Nutrition, 18*(4), 571-581. doi:http://dx.doi.org/10.1017/S1368980014002559

Neel J.V., Weder, A.B., & Julius S. (1998). Type II diabetes, essential hypertension, and obesity as "syndromes of impaired genetic homeostasis": the "thrifty genotype" hypothesis enters the 21st century. *Perspect. Biol. Med.*; 42(1):44-74.

Pontzer, H. (July 2015). Constrained total energy expenditure and the evolutionary biology of energy balance. *Exercise and Sport Sciences Reviews*, 43(3), 110-116.

Shiraev, T. & Barclay, G. (2012). Evidence based exercise: Clinical benefits of high intensity interval training. *Australian Family Physician, 41*(12): 960-2.

Swift, D. L., Johannsen, N. M., Lavie, C. J., Earnest, C. l ., & Church, T. S. (2014). The role of exercise and physical activity in weight loss and maintenance, *Progress in Cardiovascular Diseases.* (56): 441-447.

Wang, L., Liu, W., He, X., Chen, Y., Lu, J., Liu, K., . . . Yin, P. (2016). Association of overweight and obesity with patient mortality after acute myocardial infarction: A meta-analysis of prospective studies. *International Journal of Obesity, 40*(2), 220-228. doi:http://dx.doi.org/10.1038/ijo.2015.176

Acknowledgements

I'd like to thank everyone who had a hand in making this book: my wife, who understands that when I launch into a huge project, I'll be consumed; my sister who is writing her own book, which finally got me moving in that direction; and my brother who is the real writer in the family. I'd also like to thank all my initial group of testers: Christie, Cheri, Dave, Debi, Erin, Greg, Karen, Larry, Matt, Pam, and Tara.

I'd also like to thank Victoria Valentine, my book designer. Victoria's skill and talent brought the book to life.

Finally, I'd like to thank my editor and publisher, Lynda Goldman. Without Lynda's knowledge and coaching, I'd still be thinking of writing this book.

About the Author

In the fall of 2015 my vibrant, healthy, wonderful mom was diagnosed with terminal cancer. She would have only 4 months to live. During that time, my sister, a holistic health coach, and my brother, a healer, and I researched ways to restore her. But the cancer had spread too fast and had infected her entire body.

Looking at the research, I realized that there were therapies we could all do that help mitigate the chances of cancer, but you have to start early. I began to understand that the body is an open system and to understand the body, you had look at various complicated and seemingly random processes.

Soon after my mom passed, I was at my annual physical, lamenting to my physician that I could not seem to lose or even maintain my weight. He said that maybe I should get used to my heavier weight because the effort, in terms of diet and exercise, was greater than the expected results. I rejected that advice.

Instead, I used the research skills I gained completing my doctorate and did a deep dive into the diet industry. I looked at weight loss from every angle: nutrition, diet, exercise, medicine, and holistic health. My Masters' degree in systems management and my experience as a pilot and Air Force officer taught me that to be complete, the separate research towers had to be combined. This was a special skill I was born with.

My "ah ha" moment came when I realized that having weight loss as a goal put the body and mind in conflict, making weight loss less likely. My physician also relayed a story about one of his patients who had lost 180 lbs. When I asked how, he said his patient had one simple formula. He lost 2 pounds of baggage for every pound of fat lost. These are the seeds of the Ultimate diet Process. I followed the research where it led and found 8 principles that had weight loss as a side effect. Once weight is just a data point, I could happily watch the weight fall off, without effort.

That's my gift to you: the paradigm shift from everything you've heard to everything you can be. I live my life deliberately, and you can too.

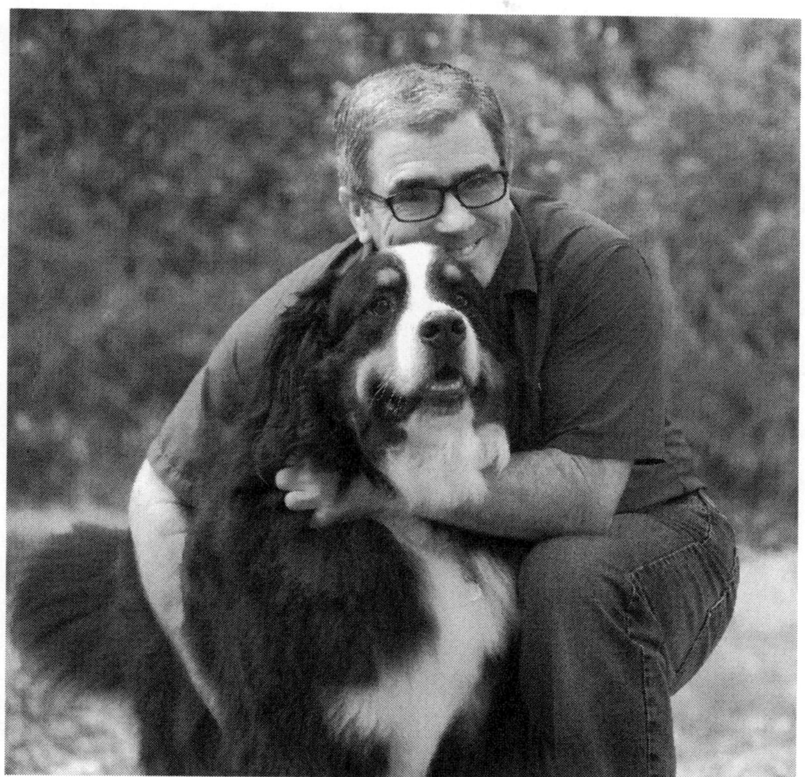

Photo by Victoria Brown

How else can I help you?

Are you looking for a speaker at your next event or conference?

Whether you're in the airline industry, or have a corporate event or sales meeting coming up, contact Dr. Michael for a motivating talk, along with copies of *2 Day Gift of Wellness* for your members or employees.

Need ongoing support?

Join our community on Facebook, and connect with people just like you who are benefitting from the UdP, with weight loss as a side effect: www.facebook.com/groups/2DayGift/

Need personal help? Find out about getting a mentor, here: www.2dayGift.com/Mentoring

And please be sure to get your two beautiful color charts, plus your journal page, by clicking here: www.2dayGift.com/gifts

You'll also receive blog posts with tips and ideas to support you on your journey to your ideal weight and best health.

To engage Dr. Michael to speak for your organization or for bulk pricing on this book, please contact

DrMichael@2dayGift.com
www.2dayGift.com

51448234R00111

Made in the USA
San Bernardino, CA
22 July 2017